21-DAY MIND DIET

PLAN FOR SENIORS OVER 60

GRAPEVINE BOOKS

Published by
GRAPEVINE BOOKS

www.grapevinebooks.com
email: contact@grapevinebooks.com

Ordering Information:
Quantity sales: Special discounts are available on quantity purchases by corporations, associations, and others.
For details, reach out to the publisher.

First published by Grapevine Books, 2025

CONTENTS

PART 1: FOUNDATIONS OF BRAIN & HEART HEALTH

1. WHAT IS THE MIND DIET? 05

2. HOW THE MIND DIET SUPPORTS BRAIN AGING 07

3. UNDERSTANDING MEMORY, FOCUS & COGNITIVE DECLINE 09

4. THE SCIENCE BEHIND ALZHEIMER'S & DEMENTIA PREVENTION 11

5. HEART HEALTH, INFLAMMATION & LONGEVITY 13

6. KEY NUTRIENTS: OMEGA-3S, ANTIOXIDANTS & HEALTHY FATS 15

PART 2: SMART EATING FOR SENIORS

7. EASY MEAL PLANNING FOR SENIORS OVER 60 17

8. PORTION CONTROL, CLEAN EATING & LOW-SODIUM LIVING 19

9. SMART SUBSTITUTIONS FOR DIETARY NEEDS 20

10. BUDGET-FRIENDLY GROCERY SHOPPING 21

11. PANTRY STAPLES FOR A BRAIN-BOOSTING KITCHEN 22

12. SIMPLE COOKING TIPS & TOOLS FOR SENIORS 23

13. HEALTHY HABITS FOR BRAIN WELLNESS, MOOD, AND LONG-TERM SUCCESS 24

14. GUIDED MEAL PLAN FOR BRAIN HEALTH 27

PART 3: BRAIN-BOOSTING BREAKFASTS

15: LEAFY GREEN OMELETS & EGG DISHES 30

16: WHOLE-GRAIN CEREALS & PORRIDGES 36

17: BERRY-BOOSTED SMOOTHIES 41

18. SIMPLE TOASTS & SPREADS WITH HEALTHY FATS 46

19. BRAINY BREAKFAST BOWLS 51

20. ON-THE-GO SENIOR-FRIENDLY MORNING MEALS 56

PART 4: NOURISHING LUNCHES & DINNERS

21. HEARTY SOUPS & STEWS FOR COGNITIVE CLARITY 61

22. POWER SALADS WITH LEAFY GREENS & NUTS 67

23. GRAIN BOWLS WITH OMEGA-3 PROTEINS 72

24. ALZHEIMER'S-FIGHTING FISH & POULTRY MEALS 77

25. PLANT-BASED MAINS FOR MOOD SUPPORT 82

26. LOW-SODIUM COMFORT FOOD CLASSICS 87

27. ONE-PAN MEALS FOR EASY CLEANUP 93

28. ANTI-INFLAMMATORY PASTA & GRAIN DISHES 98

29. LIGHT & NOURISHING DINNERS 103

30. MEMORY-BOOSTING CASSEROLES 109

PART 5: SNACKS, SIDES & SIPS

31. BRAIN-BOOSTING SNACKS 115

32. VEGGIE-BASED DIPS & SPREADS 120

33. MOOD-SUPPORTING SOUPS & SIDES 125

34. HEALTHY FATS IN QUICK BITES 130

35. SMOOTHIES, JUICES & INFUSED WATERS 135

36. SWEET TREATS WITH MEMORY BENEFITS 140

PART 6: LIFESTYLE & LONG-TERM VITALITY

37. STAYING MENTALLY SHARP BEYOND THE PLATE: DAILY ROUTINES FOR LONGEVITY & WELLNESS 145

38. GLOSSARY OF INGREDIENTS & NUTRITIONAL TERMS 147

39. FAQS ON SENIOR NUTRITION 149

40. FINAL THOUGHTS: A LONG, SHARP, INDEPENDENT LIFE 151

PART 1
FOUNDATIONS OF BRAIN & HEART HEALTH

1. WHAT IS THE MIND DIET?

Aging comes with many changes, but one of the most significant is how our brains function. Many seniors begin to notice slower recall, lapses in memory, or difficulty concentrating. While some cognitive change is normal, science shows that **what we eat can directly impact how sharp our minds stay**. That's where the **MIND diet** comes in.

The **MIND diet** stands for **Mediterranean-DASH Intervention for Neurodegenerative Delay**. It's a nutritional plan that combines two already well-known and respected diets: the **Mediterranean diet** and the **DASH diet** (Dietary Approaches to Stop Hypertension). Both of these diets are praised for improving heart health and reducing inflammation. But the MIND diet goes a step further. It focuses specifically on foods that support **brain health**, helping to preserve memory, improve focus, and potentially reduce the risk of **Alzheimer's disease** and other forms of dementia.

The MIND diet was developed by **researchers at Rush University Medical Center**, who wanted to find a simple, science-backed way to slow cognitive decline. After studying thousands of seniors, they found that individuals who followed the MIND diet closely had a **53% lower risk of developing Alzheimer's**, while those who followed it moderately still saw a **35% reduction in risk**. Those are powerful numbers. And they offer real hope to anyone who wants to protect their brain as they age.

So, what does the MIND diet actually include? The plan highlights **10 brain-healthy food groups** and limits **5 unhealthy ones**. Let's start with the good news.

The 10 foods you are encouraged to eat regularly are:

1. **Leafy green vegetables** like spinach, kale, and collards.
2. **Other vegetables**, especially colorful ones rich in antioxidants.
3. **Nuts**, which provide healthy fats and vitamin E.
4. **Berries**, particularly blueberries and strawberries, known for their brain-boosting antioxidants.
5. **Beans**, which are full of fiber and plant-based protein.
6. **Whole grains** such as brown rice, oatmeal, and quinoa.
7. **Fish**, especially fatty fish rich in **omega-3s** like salmon and sardines.
8. **Poultry**, like chicken or turkey, two or more times a week.
9. **Olive oil**, used as the primary cooking fat.
10. **Wine**, in moderation (no more than one glass per day).

Each of these foods is selected because of its nutrients, antioxidants, or healthy fats that support **brain**

function, memory retention, and **mental clarity**.

The MIND diet also recommends **limiting** the following five food groups:

1. **Red meats**
2. **Butter and stick margarine**
3. **Cheese**
4. **Pastries and sweets**
5. **Fried or fast food**

These items tend to be high in **saturated fats, trans fats**, and added sugars, which are linked to increased **inflammation**, **oxidative stress**, and faster cognitive decline.

What makes the MIND diet especially senior-friendly is its simplicity. It's not about counting calories or eliminating entire food groups. Instead, it offers a **flexible, manageable framework** based on foods you likely already enjoy. For example, just adding a handful of berries to your breakfast or using olive oil instead of butter on vegetables can have measurable effects over time.

Another benefit? The MIND diet is also great for your **heart health**. Since it includes many anti-inflammatory and antioxidant-rich ingredients, it supports overall wellness, not just mental clarity. In fact, many experts consider the brain and heart to be deeply connected, meaning what's good for your heart is almost always good for your brain too.

For those over 60, this becomes even more important. As we age, our risk for chronic conditions like **hypertension, diabetes**, and **stroke** increases. These conditions also raise the risk for dementia and cognitive impairment. By choosing foods that stabilize blood pressure, improve circulation, and reduce plaque buildup in arteries, you are protecting both your body and your mind.

Now, what about the **emotional benefits** of this way of eating? People who follow the MIND diet often report better moods, more energy, and less mental fog. The nutrients in berries, greens, and fatty fish can influence neurotransmitter production, such as serotonin and dopamine, which play a key role in mood regulation. Simply put, eating well helps you feel more like yourself again.

The MIND diet is not a fad or a short-term cleanse. It's a long-term lifestyle approach to **slow aging** and support **mental sharpness**. And the best part is that it doesn't require perfection. Even those who follow it "most of the time" still see meaningful benefits. It's not about doing everything right. It's about making **better choices more often**.

In this cookbook, you'll find **easy recipes using simple ingredients**, many of them with only five components. Each dish is designed to fit into the MIND diet guidelines without requiring exotic ingredients or hours in the kitchen. Whether you're cooking for yourself, your spouse, or your grandchildren, you'll find meals that are both delicious and deeply nourishing.

The takeaway is simple. **You have more control over your brain health than you think.** And the MIND diet is a powerful, proven way to support that goal—one meal at a time.

2. HOW THE MIND DIET SUPPORTS BRAIN AGING

Aging is natural, but how we age can look very different from person to person. Some people remain mentally sharp into their 80s and 90s. Others begin to notice changes in memory, thinking, or focus much earlier. While genetics play a role, research now shows that **diet is one of the most powerful tools we have to protect brain function** as we grow older.

The **MIND diet** was developed to target this exact need. Unlike trendy diets that focus on weight loss or short-term results, the MIND diet is based on years of scientific research. It was designed specifically to reduce the risk of **neurodegenerative diseases** like **Alzheimer's** and to help the brain stay healthy throughout the aging process.

So, how exactly does it work?

The answer lies in the way food interacts with the brain. Our brains are made up of billions of neurons. These cells communicate using chemical signals and require constant fuel to function properly. As we age, these cells can become damaged by **oxidative stress**, **inflammation**, and **poor blood flow**. The MIND diet helps slow this process by offering the brain the nutrients it needs and avoiding the substances that can cause harm.

The key idea behind the MIND diet is to **feed the brain with protective compounds**. These include **antioxidants**, **healthy fats**, **vitamins**, and **anti-inflammatory nutrients**. Foods like **berries, leafy greens, olive oil, nuts, and fatty fish** are rich in these compounds. When eaten regularly, they help reduce damage to brain cells and support new brain cell growth.

Let's take **oxidative stress**, for example. This happens when unstable molecules, called free radicals, build up in the body and start damaging cells. Over time, this damage affects the brain's ability to function, leading to memory loss and slower thinking. The MIND diet is rich in **antioxidants**, which neutralize free radicals and prevent this type of cellular harm.

Another common issue with aging brains is **inflammation**. Chronic inflammation has been linked to cognitive decline, mood disorders, and dementia. Many of the foods encouraged in the MIND diet—such as berries, olive oil, and nuts—are **anti-inflammatory**, meaning they help cool down the body's stress response and protect delicate brain tissue.

The MIND diet also supports **better blood flow to the brain**. Whole grains, fish, and greens help keep arteries flexible and clear. This ensures that the brain receives plenty of oxygen and nutrients. A well-nourished brain is more resilient and better able to adapt to the changes that come with age.

Perhaps one of the most exciting effects of the MIND diet is its impact on **memory and learning**. In a major study conducted by researchers at Rush University, seniors who followed the MIND diet closely showed a much **slower rate of cognitive decline** than those who did not. In fact, their brains functioned as if they were **7.5 years younger**. That is not just a small benefit. That is life-changing.

The MIND diet does not just help with memory. It also supports **focus, mental clarity, and emotional balance**. That is because many of its recommended foods contain compounds that influence brain chemicals like **serotonin and dopamine**. These chemicals affect how we feel, think, and respond to stress. By eating foods that support their production, seniors may experience **less anxiety, better mood, and a more stable sense of well-being**.

In addition to these direct effects, the MIND diet also helps with conditions that indirectly affect brain aging. For example, **high blood pressure, high cholesterol, and type 2 diabetes** all increase the risk of dementia. The MIND diet's focus on **whole foods and healthy fats** can help regulate blood sugar, lower cholesterol, and maintain healthy blood pressure levels. This reduces overall risk and keeps both the body and brain working better for longer.

One of the best things about the MIND diet is that it is not rigid or overwhelming. Seniors do not need to become perfect eaters to enjoy the benefits. Even moderate adherence to the diet has been shown to make a meaningful difference in brain health. You do not need to change everything overnight. Simply adding more leafy greens, cutting back on processed foods, and swapping butter for olive oil are steps in the right direction.

The MIND diet also encourages regularity. The brain thrives on consistency. By eating brain-healthy foods daily—not just once in a while—you create habits that help protect the brain over time. Think of it like maintenance. Just as you would maintain a car or a home, you can maintain your brain with the right fuel.

Lastly, it is worth noting that the MIND diet is also a **hopeful approach**. It does not dwell on fear. Instead, it empowers seniors to take action. You are not powerless in the face of aging. You can choose meals that help you stay alert, independent, and mentally strong.

In this cookbook, you will find a wide variety of recipes that align with the MIND diet principles. These meals are not only healthy but also enjoyable. You will be able to care for your brain without giving up the pleasure of food. And that is the true beauty of the MIND diet—it supports your mind while honoring your life.

3. UNDERSTANDING MEMORY, FOCUS & COGNITIVE DECLINE

Have you ever walked into a room and forgotten why you went there? Or struggled to remember someone's name even though you just met them last week? These moments can feel frustrating or even scary. But they are also common, especially as we age. To care for our brains properly, it helps to understand what is really happening with **memory, focus, and cognitive decline**.

Our brains are incredibly complex. They store every experience, process every thought, and guide every action. But just like the rest of our bodies, the brain changes over time. Some forgetfulness is a **normal part of aging**, and not every lapse is a sign of something serious. Still, recognizing the difference between normal aging and concerning cognitive decline is important for long-term brain health.

Memory is the brain's ability to store and retrieve information. There are several types of memory, but the most affected by age are **short-term memory** and **working memory**. Short-term memory helps us remember things for a few seconds or minutes, like a phone number we just heard. Working memory allows us to hold and manipulate information in our minds, like remembering a set of directions while driving. As we grow older, it can take longer to recall certain details or organize thoughts clearly. This is often due to **slower communication between brain cells** and less efficient processing.

Focus, on the other hand, is our ability to pay attention to what matters. Good focus helps us complete tasks, follow conversations, and make decisions. As attention weakens with age, we might find ourselves feeling more distracted or overwhelmed in noisy or busy environments. This can make everyday situations—like reading a recipe or having a group conversation—more difficult. The good news is that focus, like memory, can be supported and strengthened through daily habits and nutrition.

When these mental functions begin to decline more rapidly than expected, we enter the territory of **cognitive decline**. This can range from mild cognitive impairment, where a person notices subtle changes in memory and thinking, to serious conditions like **dementia and Alzheimer's disease**. Cognitive decline is not a normal part of aging. It signals that the brain is no longer functioning as well as it should.

Many factors influence whether or not someone experiences cognitive decline. Some of them, like genetics and age, are out of our control. But others—including **diet, exercise, sleep, and mental stimulation**—can be improved at any time in life. Research shows that **lifestyle choices play a major role in maintaining brain function**. What we eat, how we move, and even how we manage stress can either protect the brain or put it at risk.

So how does **nutrition** come into play?

The brain is one of the most energy-demanding organs in the body. It requires a steady supply of oxygen, nutrients, and healthy fats to function at its best. When we give it what it needs, we support memory, attention, and mood. When we feed it processed foods, unhealthy fats, and too much sugar, we increase inflammation and oxidative stress. These are two of the biggest enemies of brain health.

Inflammation in the brain can interfere with communication between neurons. This may show up as forgetfulness, slower thinking, or trouble concentrating. **Oxidative stress**, caused by unstable molecules called free radicals, can damage brain cells over time. Foods that are rich in **antioxidants**—such as berries, leafy greens, and nuts—help protect the brain from this kind of damage.

Poor **blood flow** is another major contributor to cognitive decline. Conditions like high blood pressure and high cholesterol can reduce circulation to the brain, depriving it of vital nutrients. Diets that are high in sodium, sugar, and unhealthy fats worsen this effect. On the flip side, foods like salmon, whole grains, olive oil, and legumes help **support healthy circulation** and protect the brain from deterioration.

What about mental sharpness? Memory and focus are not just about brain chemistry. They also depend on how we use our brains. Seniors who stay mentally engaged—by reading, solving puzzles, trying new skills, or learning something new—often report **better memory and attention** than those who are less active. When combined with brain-friendly foods, this kind of mental stimulation acts like a workout for the mind.

Another important factor is **mood**. Depression, anxiety, and loneliness can all affect memory and cognitive performance. Seniors who feel isolated or sad may find it harder to focus, recall information, or feel motivated. A healthy diet, along with regular physical activity and social engagement, can significantly improve emotional health and cognitive outlook.

The MIND diet was created with all of these insights in mind. By focusing on **brain-boosting nutrients**, **anti-inflammatory foods**, and **simple eating habits**, it offers a practical way to protect memory and preserve mental clarity. You do not need to understand every chemical process or memorize complex health theories. You simply need to make better food choices, one meal at a time.

Memory, focus, and clear thinking are not just nice to have. They are essential for living fully and independently. By understanding what drives cognitive decline and taking steps to protect your brain today, you are investing in a healthier, sharper tomorrow.

4. THE SCIENCE BEHIND ALZHEIMER'S & DEMENTIA PREVENTION

Alzheimer's disease and dementia are among the most feared conditions associated with aging. They affect not only memory and thinking but also independence, relationships, and quality of life. But here's the hopeful truth. Scientists now believe that many cases of Alzheimer's and dementia can be delayed, and in some cases, even prevented, through simple changes in lifestyle. One of the most powerful tools? **What we eat.**

To understand how prevention works, it helps to first understand what these diseases are. **Alzheimer's disease** is the most common form of dementia, a group of disorders that affect memory, reasoning, and behavior. It slowly destroys brain cells and interferes with daily life. While it is more common in people over 65, it is not a normal part of aging. **Dementia** is a broader term that includes Alzheimer's, as well as conditions like vascular dementia and Lewy body dementia.

At the heart of Alzheimer's is the buildup of **abnormal proteins in the brain**. These proteins, called **amyloid plaques** and **tau tangles**, interrupt the brain's communication pathways. As they spread, they damage brain cells and shrink vital areas responsible for memory, decision-making, and self-control. Eventually, this leads to confusion, mood changes, memory loss, and a loss of independence.

So what causes these protein buildups to start? That's where the science gets interesting. Researchers have found that **inflammation, oxidative stress, poor blood flow**, and **insulin resistance** all play major roles. These are not random problems. They are often linked to long-term lifestyle patterns, especially diet and exercise.

Let's break these factors down.

Inflammation is the body's natural response to injury or infection. But when it becomes chronic, it can damage healthy tissue, including the brain. Diets high in processed foods, sugar, and saturated fats can trigger ongoing inflammation. On the other hand, foods rich in **antioxidants and omega-3 fats**—like berries, leafy greens, nuts, and salmon—help calm inflammation and protect brain cells.

Oxidative stress happens when unstable molecules called **free radicals** build up and begin to harm cells. The brain, because of its high oxygen use, is especially vulnerable. Antioxidants from foods like blueberries, spinach, and dark chocolate help neutralize these molecules and reduce damage.

Another key factor is **blood flow to the brain**. Just like your heart, your brain needs a steady supply of oxygen and nutrients to function. High blood pressure, high cholesterol, and narrowed arteries can reduce circulation and starve the brain. Over time, this leads to the loss of mental sharpness. The MIND diet promotes foods that support healthy blood vessels, such as whole grains, legumes, and olive oil.

Insulin resistance—a condition often seen in type 2 diabetes—can also increase the risk of Alzheimer's. Insulin helps brain cells absorb glucose, their primary fuel. When cells become resistant to insulin, energy production slows and the brain suffers. Diets that are low in refined sugars and high in fiber can help regulate blood sugar and reduce this risk.

There is also growing evidence that **gut health** plays a role in brain health. The gut and brain communicate through a network called the **gut-brain axis**. Inflammation or imbalance in gut bacteria can affect mood, memory, and cognition. Fiber-rich foods, probiotics, and a diverse plant-based diet all support a healthier gut and, in turn, a healthier brain.

Now let's look at what this means in real life. In long-term studies, seniors who followed a **MIND diet** were found to have a significantly **lower risk of developing Alzheimer's disease**. One major study from Rush University showed that seniors who closely followed the MIND diet had a **53 percent lower risk**, and even moderate followers saw a **35 percent reduction**. These results are exciting because they show that **even partial adherence helps**.

The MIND diet combines the best elements of the **Mediterranean** and **DASH diets**, both of which have long been known to support heart and brain health. But the MIND diet goes further by emphasizing foods most closely tied to cognitive protection. These include **berries, leafy greens, nuts, whole grains, fish, poultry, olive oil**, and a limited amount of wine. It also recommends **avoiding red meats, fried foods, butter, cheese**, and sweets.

Prevention is not about perfection. It is about **small, consistent changes** that support brain health over time. You don't need to become a nutrition expert to make a difference. Swapping out white bread for whole grain, adding a few servings of vegetables to your week, or replacing butter with olive oil can all reduce your long-term risk.

The truth is, many people wait until they notice memory problems before taking action. But the best time to protect your brain is **before symptoms begin**. Alzheimer's can develop silently for years. Prevention starts today, with the choices you make at the table.

This cookbook gives you the tools to build those habits. With **easy recipes, familiar ingredients**, and a focus on **brain-boosting foods**, you will find it easier than ever to eat in a way that supports your mind. And the science agrees—what you eat matters. You can take control of your brain health, one meal at a time.

5. HEART HEALTH, INFLAMMATION & LONGEVITY

The heart and brain may seem like two separate organs, but they are deeply connected. What keeps your heart strong also protects your brain. In fact, when your heart is healthy, your brain receives more oxygen and nutrients, making it easier to think clearly, stay focused, and remember important details. As we age, taking care of both becomes essential for a long and independent life.

Let us start with the heart. This powerful muscle beats more than 100,000 times a day, pumping blood to every part of the body. That includes the brain, which uses around 20 percent of the body's oxygen supply. When the heart struggles—due to clogged arteries, high blood pressure, or poor circulation—the brain suffers too. Over time, poor heart health can lead to memory loss, confusion, and even increase the risk of dementia.

The MIND diet, originally developed to slow cognitive decline, also offers **major benefits for heart health**. It encourages foods that reduce **cholesterol, lower blood pressure**, and support **healthy circulation**. These include **leafy greens, nuts, berries, whole grains, olive oil, beans**, and **fish**. These ingredients are rich in vitamins, minerals, fiber, and healthy fats that help the heart work efficiently.

A major threat to both heart and brain is **inflammation**. While inflammation is the body's natural response to injury or infection, it becomes dangerous when it turns chronic. Long-term inflammation damages blood vessels, stiffens arteries, and creates stress throughout the body. It is closely linked to **heart disease, stroke**, and **Alzheimer's**.

What causes this type of inflammation? Often, it comes from poor diet. Foods high in **trans fats, refined sugar, processed meat**, and **excess sodium** trigger the body's inflammatory response. Over time, this damages tissues and organs, especially the heart and brain.

The MIND diet helps calm this response by offering **anti-inflammatory foods**. Berries are packed with antioxidants. Leafy greens provide vitamin K, folate, and fiber. Olive oil contains healthy fats that soothe inflammation in the arteries. Even a handful of walnuts or a serving of salmon can reduce the markers of inflammation in your bloodstream.

But inflammation is not only a physical problem. It is also tied to **emotional health**. Chronic inflammation can increase the risk of depression, anxiety, and fatigue. These conditions affect motivation, sleep, and even appetite. When you feel mentally and emotionally drained, it becomes harder to stick to healthy habits. By reducing inflammation, you not only support your body but also improve your mood and mental clarity.

Another benefit of the MIND diet is how it helps **regulate blood pressure**. High blood pressure, also called hypertension, is often called the silent killer because it rarely has symptoms. But its impact is serious. It forces the heart to work harder and damages the arteries. It also increases the risk of stroke and brain damage. The MIND diet's focus on potassium-rich foods like spinach, beans, and bananas can help maintain a healthy balance of fluids and support healthy blood pressure.

Heart health is also linked to **cholesterol levels**. LDL cholesterol, often called the "bad" cholesterol, can build up in the arteries and block blood flow. HDL cholesterol, the "good" kind, helps clear this buildup. The MIND diet promotes the increase of HDL and reduction of LDL by encouraging healthy fats and cutting back on saturated fats. Replacing butter with olive oil, choosing fish over red meat, and eating more fiber-rich foods can all improve cholesterol levels.

Now let us talk about **longevity**. Living longer is not just about adding years to your life. It is about adding life to your years. That means staying active, thinking clearly, and feeling strong well into your 70s, 80s, and beyond. Diet plays a huge role in this. People who follow heart-healthy, anti-inflammatory diets tend to live longer and enjoy a higher quality of life.

Studies have shown that seniors who eat more **plant-based, whole foods** and fewer processed items have lower rates of heart disease, diabetes, and stroke. They also experience fewer hospital visits and take fewer medications. That means more freedom, more energy, and more time spent doing what they love.

Longevity is also supported by healthy habits outside the kitchen. Regular physical activity, quality sleep, stress management, and strong social connections all contribute to a longer, happier life. But diet is the foundation. You eat multiple times a day. Every meal is a chance to support your heart and your future.

The beauty of the MIND diet is that it is simple, flexible, and satisfying. You do not need to count every calorie or give up everything you enjoy. Instead, you build meals around ingredients that love you back. You swap, not sacrifice. And you make choices that strengthen your heart, protect your brain, and set you up for a longer, fuller life.

This cookbook gives you the tools to begin. With every recipe, you will be making progress toward a healthier heart, a clearer mind, and a longer, more vibrant life. It is never too late to take control of your health. Start today, and let your meals become your medicine.

6. KEY NUTRIENTS: OMEGA-3S, ANTIOXIDANTS & HEALTHY FATS

When it comes to protecting the brain and heart as we age, not all nutrients are created equal. Some foods simply have more power than others. Among the most important nutrients for brain health and longevity are **omega-3 fatty acids, antioxidants**, and **healthy fats**. These three groups of nutrients work together to reduce inflammation, protect cells from damage, and support sharp thinking well into your golden years.

Let us start with **omega-3 fatty acids**. These are essential fats that your body cannot produce on its own. That means you must get them from your diet. Omega-3s are found in high amounts in **fatty fish** such as salmon, sardines, mackerel, and trout. Plant-based sources include **chia seeds, flaxseeds, walnuts**, and algae-based supplements.

So why are omega-3s important? These fats are critical for **building and repairing brain cells**. They help keep the outer layer of brain cells flexible and efficient, which improves communication between neurons. Better communication leads to better memory, faster thinking, and improved focus. Studies show that seniors who eat omega-3-rich foods regularly have a lower risk of **cognitive decline, dementia**, and even **depression**.

Omega-3s also reduce **inflammation** throughout the body. Chronic inflammation is a major cause of heart disease and has been linked to Alzheimer's and other forms of dementia. By eating more omega-3s, you help your body fight back against this invisible damage.

Another benefit of omega-3s is their effect on **mood and mental well-being**. These fats support the production of important brain chemicals like serotonin and dopamine, which help regulate emotions. Seniors who consume more omega-3s often report better mood stability, less anxiety, and a more positive outlook on life.

Next, let us talk about **antioxidants**. These powerful compounds protect the body from something called **oxidative stress**. This stress happens when unstable molecules known as **free radicals** build up in the body and start attacking healthy cells. The brain is especially vulnerable to this kind of damage, partly because it uses a lot of oxygen and has a high fat content.

Antioxidants **neutralize free radicals** and prevent them from doing harm. They are found in a wide variety of colorful fruits and vegetables, especially those with deep, rich colors. Some of the best sources include **blueberries, strawberries, spinach, kale, beets, carrots**, and **bell peppers**. Green tea, dark chocolate, and certain herbs and spices like turmeric also contain strong antioxidant properties.

What makes antioxidants so powerful for aging brains is their ability to **protect memory, delay cognitive decline**, and reduce damage to brain tissue. In long-term studies, people who eat more antioxidant-rich foods perform better on memory tests and are less likely to develop dementia.

Antioxidants also support **immune health**, reduce inflammation, and help protect the heart. That is why the MIND diet includes so many antioxidant-packed ingredients in every meal. Whether you are eating a salad full of leafy greens or a bowl of mixed berries, you are fueling your body with brain-loving compounds that support clear thinking and long-term wellness.

Now let us focus on **healthy fats**. Not all fats are bad. In fact, some are absolutely necessary. Your brain is made up of about 60 percent fat. It needs the right kinds of fats to stay flexible, well-nourished, and responsive. Healthy fats also support the heart by improving cholesterol levels, reducing blood pressure, and supporting healthy blood flow.

The best sources of healthy fats include **extra virgin olive oil, avocados, nuts, seeds**, and **fatty fish**. These fats provide energy, help absorb vitamins, and protect against inflammation. Olive oil, in particular, is a cornerstone of the MIND diet. It is used for cooking, dressings, and even drizzling over vegetables. Just one tablespoon a day has been shown to improve heart health and reduce markers of inflammation.

Avocados are another smart choice. They are full of **monounsaturated fats**, which help lower LDL cholesterol and raise HDL cholesterol—the kind that protects your arteries. Plus, they are rich in potassium, fiber, and vitamin E, all of which support brain and heart function.

Nuts like **walnuts, almonds, and pistachios** are also full of healthy fats and provide a satisfying crunch that makes meals more enjoyable. A handful of nuts a few times a week can support memory, reduce the risk of heart disease, and help keep blood sugar levels stable.

When you include these nutrients—**omega-3s, antioxidants, and healthy fats**—in your daily meals, you are giving your body exactly what it needs to age well. These nutrients do not just add years to your life. They add clarity, vitality, and energy to your day.

Eating for brain health is not about strict rules or complicated plans. It is about choosing foods that give your body the tools to repair, protect, and thrive. With every meal, you have a chance to nourish your brain, support your heart, and strengthen your future.

In the recipes that follow, you will see how easy it is to include these key nutrients. Whether you are enjoying a berry smoothie, a spinach salad with olive oil, or a salmon dinner, you are doing more than just eating. You are investing in a longer, healthier, and more vibrant life.

PART 2

SMART EATING FOR SENIORS

7. EASY MEAL PLANNING FOR SENIORS OVER 60

As we grow older, the way we eat matters more than ever. The right meals can help keep your brain sharp, your heart strong, and your body full of energy. But planning those meals can sometimes feel overwhelming. You might wonder where to start, what to buy, or how to cook something healthy that still tastes good. The good news is that **meal planning can be simple, stress-free, and even enjoyable**.

Meal planning is not about following a strict diet or spending hours in the kitchen. It is about making life easier and more organized. For seniors over 60, the focus should be on **nutritious, balanced meals** that are easy to prepare and gentle on digestion. That means choosing foods that support your brain, heart, and joints, while avoiding anything that causes inflammation, fatigue, or brain fog.

The first step is to **set a routine**. A basic weekly plan can take away the daily guesswork. Start by choosing just three meals a day and maybe one small snack. Think about your favorite foods and find ways to include brain-boosting ingredients like **berries, leafy greens, olive oil, whole grains, beans, fish**, and **nuts**. These staples of the MIND diet are easy to mix and match in different combinations.

Next, make a simple **grocery list**. Focus on whole foods and ingredients that can be used in multiple recipes. For example, spinach can go into omelets, soups, and salads. Oats can be used for breakfast or even in baked snacks. Salmon can be grilled for dinner and turned into a sandwich the next day. Buying foods that serve more than one purpose saves money and time.

Batch cooking is another helpful strategy. Try preparing two or three meals in advance and storing them in the fridge or freezer. This works especially well for soups, stews, casseroles, and roasted vegetables. On days when you feel tired or busy, you will have a healthy option ready to go. That means fewer last-minute decisions and less temptation to reach for processed or sugary foods.

If cooking every day feels like too much, consider **rotating meals**. Choose a few breakfast options, a few lunches, and a few dinners that you enjoy. Then repeat them each week with slight variations. For example, one week you might have oatmeal with berries, and the next week you switch to a berry smoothie. You are still getting the same nutrients, but with enough variety to keep things interesting.

Do not forget about **portion control**. As metabolism slows with age, the body needs fewer calories but more nutrients. That means focusing on quality over quantity. Fill your plate with vegetables, lean proteins, healthy fats, and fiber-rich carbs. A smaller serving of a nutrient-dense meal is better than a large plate of empty calories.

Another helpful habit is **writing your plan down**. Use a notepad or calendar to jot down what you will eat each day. This visual guide makes shopping and cooking easier and removes the stress of making decisions on the spot. It also helps you track which meals you liked and which ones you want to change.

When planning meals, always consider **your specific health needs**. If you are managing diabetes, high blood pressure, or digestive issues, adjust recipes accordingly. Use low-sodium ingredients, avoid added sugars, and focus on high-fiber foods. The MIND diet is naturally supportive of most health conditions, but personalizing it makes it even more effective.

Keep cooking tools and kitchen setup in mind too. Make sure your space is safe and easy to use. Place commonly used ingredients and utensils within reach. Consider using lightweight pots, sharp peelers, or kitchen tools designed for seniors with limited hand strength or arthritis. A well-organized kitchen makes cooking feel less like a chore and more like an enjoyable routine.

One overlooked aspect of meal planning is **hydration**. Many seniors do not drink enough water during the day, which can lead to fatigue, confusion, and even poor appetite. Aim to drink water regularly and include hydrating foods like cucumbers, melons, soups, and herbal teas in your meal plan.

Lastly, do not feel like you have to do everything alone. If you have a partner, family member, or caregiver, involve them in your meal planning. Share your favorite recipes, prep meals together, or take turns cooking. If you live alone, look into local programs that deliver healthy meals for seniors. The goal is to create a sustainable routine that supports your health and fits your lifestyle.

Meal planning is not about perfection. It is about making life easier, one meal at a time. With just a little preparation each week, you can enjoy **nutritious, brain-friendly meals** without stress or confusion. The more you plan, the more control you gain over your health, your time, and your peace of mind.

Your brain and body deserve nourishment. And it does not have to be complicated. With a few smart habits, you can eat well, feel better, and enjoy your golden years with clarity and strength.

8. PORTION CONTROL, CLEAN EATING & LOW-SODIUM LIVING

Have you ever finished a meal and realized you ate more than you meant to? Or grabbed a frozen dinner only to discover it had nearly a whole day's worth of sodium? It happens. But small changes in how we eat can make a big difference, especially after 60.

Let's start with **portion control**. As we age, our bodies need fewer calories but more nutrients. That means it's not about eating less. It's about eating smarter. Try using smaller plates. Slow down while eating. Listen to your body. Are you full, or just finishing what's in front of you? Learning to stop when you're satisfied helps avoid overeating and supports digestion.

Now, what exactly is **clean eating**? It's simpler than it sounds. Clean eating means choosing foods that are as close to their natural state as possible. Think fresh vegetables, fruits, whole grains, lean proteins, and healthy fats. It means fewer boxed meals, fewer mystery ingredients, and more real food. Your body knows what to do with a sweet potato. It may not recognize half the ingredients in a snack bar.

And finally, there's **low-sodium living**. Did you know that too much salt can raise blood pressure and stress your heart and brain? Most sodium sneaks in through canned soups, deli meats, frozen meals, and restaurant food. The good news is that your taste buds adjust. When you start seasoning with herbs, garlic, lemon, or vinegar instead of salt, you begin to enjoy flavors in a whole new way.

You do not need to overhaul your diet overnight. Begin by reading labels. Swap one processed item for something fresh. Cook at home a little more often. Every small change adds up.

Eating well after 60 is not about restriction. It's about intention. Choose foods that love you back, and your body will thank you with better energy, clearer thinking, and stronger health for the years ahead.

9. SMART SUBSTITUTIONS FOR DIETARY NEEDS

Swap your way to better health!

Simple changes, big results. Try these easy upgrades:

Instead of butter

Try **olive oil** or **mashed avocado**

Instead of white rice

Try **quinoa** or **brown rice**

Instead of regular pasta

Try **whole wheat** or **lentil pasta**

Instead of chips

Try **unsalted nuts** or **air-popped popcorn**

Instead of canned soups

Try **homemade veggie broth** or **low-sodium options**

Instead of salad dressings loaded with sugar

Try **olive oil, lemon juice**, and **herbs**

Instead of whole milk

Try **unsweetened almond, oat**, or **soy milk**

Instead of sugary desserts

Try **fresh berries** with **plain yogurt** or **baked apples with cinnamon**

Instead of store-bought sauces

Try **homemade tomato sauce** with garlic and basil

Instead of deli meats

Try **grilled chicken** or **roasted turkey slices**

These swaps are tasty, senior-friendly, and perfect for **brain and heart health**.

Eat smart. Feel better. Live fully.

10. BUDGET-FRIENDLY GROCERY SHOPPING

Eating healthy does not have to mean spending a lot. With a little planning, you can shop smarter, waste less, and still fill your plate with **nutritious, brain-boosting foods**. It all starts with a list and a strategy.

Before heading to the store, take inventory of what you already have. Then make a **grocery list based on meals you plan to cook**. This helps you avoid impulse buys and keeps your cart focused on what you actually need.

Stick to the **outer edges of the store**, where you will find fresh produce, whole grains, and lean proteins. These are the staples of the **MIND diet**. The center aisles are often packed with processed items that cost more and do less for your health.

Buy **seasonal fruits and vegetables**. They are often cheaper, fresher, and more flavorful. Frozen fruits and veggies are also great options. They are picked at peak ripeness and are just as nutritious, often at a lower price.

Buy in bulk when it makes sense. Items like oats, brown rice, dried beans, and nuts store well and can save you money over time. Just make sure you will use them before they go bad.

Choose **store-brand items** instead of name brands. They often contain the same ingredients but cost much less. Check labels to compare.

Limit packaged snacks and sugary drinks. Not only are they expensive, but they also take up space that could go to healthier items.

Shop with a full stomach. This may sound small, but hungry shoppers are more likely to make unnecessary purchases.

Use **discount cards, coupons**, or senior discounts where available. Every bit of savings helps.

Healthy eating on a budget is possible. With just a few smart habits, you can stock your kitchen with meals that support your mind, body, and wallet. Plan ahead, shop with purpose, and enjoy the peace of knowing you are eating well without overspending.

11. PANTRY STAPLES FOR A BRAIN-BOOSTING KITCHEN

Want to make healthy meals easier and faster? It all starts with a well-stocked pantry. When your kitchen is filled with the right ingredients, cooking for brain and heart health becomes simple and enjoyable.

Here are the must-have **pantry staples** every brain-boosting kitchen needs:

Whole Grains

Keep brown rice, quinoa, steel-cut oats, and whole wheat pasta on hand. These grains are packed with fiber and help keep blood sugar steady.

Canned Beans

Black beans, chickpeas, lentils, and kidney beans are rich in protein and fiber. They are perfect for soups, salads, and stews.

Nuts and Seeds

Walnuts, almonds, flaxseeds, chia seeds, and sunflower seeds support brain health with healthy fats and antioxidants. Store them in airtight containers for freshness.

Healthy Oils

Extra virgin olive oil is a staple for dressings, sautés, and roasting. It is a key part of the MIND diet and supports heart health too.

Low-Sodium Broth

Vegetable or chicken broth makes cooking easier and adds flavor without the salt.

Herbs and Spices

Turmeric, cinnamon, garlic powder, rosemary, thyme, and black pepper add flavor and fight inflammation. They also make low-salt meals more exciting.

Canned Tomatoes

Great for sauces, soups, and stews. Look for no-salt-added versions when possible.

Tinned Fish

Sardines and salmon are rich in omega-3s and easy to add to salads or grain bowls.

Nut Butters

Natural peanut or almond butter is a good source of healthy fats and protein. Check the label to avoid added sugar and salt.

Dried Fruit

A little goes a long way. Keep dried cranberries or raisins on hand to sprinkle into oatmeal or salads for a brain-friendly boost.

When your pantry is ready, cooking becomes less stressful and more nourishing. You do not need to buy everything at once. Just start adding one or two brain-healthy staples each week. Before long, you will have everything you need to create delicious, simple meals that support your mind and body.

12. SIMPLE COOKING TIPS & TOOLS FOR SENIORS

Cooking at home does not have to be complicated. In fact, with the right tools and a few smart habits, preparing healthy meals can be quick, safe, and even enjoyable. Whether you are cooking for one or two, or just looking for less effort in the kitchen, these tips will help you stay confident and stress-free.

Keep it simple.

Start with easy recipes that use a small number of ingredients. Look for meals with five ingredients or fewer. Focus on whole foods like vegetables, grains, beans, and lean proteins. You do not need gourmet skills to eat well. A simple stir-fry or soup can offer all the nutrients your brain and heart need.

Use time-saving tools.

A few kitchen gadgets can make life easier. A **slow cooker** is great for set-it-and-forget-it meals. A **microwave steamer** makes vegetables in minutes. A **small food processor** can chop onions, garlic, or herbs without tiring your hands. Nonstick pans are helpful for easier cleanup, and **lightweight cookware** is safer for lifting and moving.

Organize your kitchen.

Keep your most-used items within easy reach. Place spices, utensils, and pantry staples in spots that do not require bending or stretching. Store heavy pots at waist height to avoid injury. Use labels or clear containers so ingredients are easy to find.

Stay safe.

Sharp knives can be safer than dull ones, as they require less pressure. Use cutting boards with non-slip grips. Choose **measuring cups with large print** if you have vision concerns. If grip strength is limited, try tools with large, easy-to-hold handles.

Prep ahead.

Chop vegetables, cook grains, or portion out snacks in advance. Store extras in the fridge or freezer. This makes cooking each day faster and less tiring.

Keep it fun.

Play music, invite a friend to help, or cook with a loved one. The goal is not just healthy meals, but joy in the process.

Smart tools and simple habits make all the difference. With a bit of planning, cooking can become one of the most empowering parts of your day. You are not just feeding your body. You are caring for your mind, your heart, and your independence.

13. HEALTHY HABITS FOR BRAIN WELLNESS, MOOD, AND LONG-TERM SUCCESS

Eating well is essential, but the path to long-term brain and heart health involves more than what's on your plate. For seniors over 60, daily habits can make a huge difference in supporting memory, focus, emotional balance, and overall vitality. This chapter is your guide to living with energy, clarity, and peace of mind—every single day.

As we age, lifestyle choices affect how we feel, think, and move. A few simple routines can help slow aging, boost mental sharpness, and promote mood support. You don't need a complicated plan. Just small, steady changes that help your brain and body thrive.

Move Your Body, Feed Your Brain

Regular physical activity increases blood flow to the brain, enhancing oxygen delivery and supporting memory and focus. Even light movement, like a 20-minute walk, gardening, or gentle stretching, can help with mood, attention, and overall wellness. The key is consistency. Move in a way that feels good—daily if possible.

Get Deep, Restorative Sleep

Poor sleep affects concentration, emotional stability, and long-term brain health. Try to go to bed and wake up at the same time each day. Limit caffeine after lunch, avoid screens before bed, and keep your room cool and quiet. Rest is the body's way of resetting, healing, and preparing for another day of vitality.

Stay Mentally Engaged

Your brain craves stimulation. Read books, do puzzles, play music, or try something new. Learning strengthens cognitive clarity and builds new neural pathways, even later in life. A curious mind is a sharper mind.

Build Strong Social Connections

Loneliness and isolation can affect brain function and mood. Make regular phone calls, write letters, join a group, or visit a neighbor. Even brief interactions can improve emotional wellness and provide a powerful boost to cognitive health.

Manage Stress with Intention

Chronic stress contributes to inflammation and cognitive decline. Use tools like deep breathing, nature walks, or meditation. Gratitude journaling and prayer can also center your thoughts and lift your mood. Just a few minutes a day helps calm the mind and promote clarity.

Drink More Water

Hydration is often overlooked. Dehydration can cause fatigue, confusion, and lack of focus. Aim for 6–8 glasses daily. Add cucumber, mint, or lemon for extra brain-boosting benefits.

Focus on Purpose and Joy

Having a reason to get up in the morning—no matter how small—improves emotional resilience and supports healthy brain chemistry. Purpose can come from hobbies, helping others, learning something new, or simply enjoying your morning tea with gratitude.

Top 10 Foods for Mood, Vitality, and Mental Wellness

These nutrient-rich ingredients help support mood stability, emotional wellness, brain function, and slow aging naturally:

1. **Blueberries** – Packed with antioxidants that support memory and reduce brain fog
2. **Leafy Greens** – Kale, spinach, and chard help fight inflammation and support cognitive clarity
3. **Salmon** – High in omega-3s to protect brain cells and boost mood-regulating hormones
4. **Walnuts** – A perfect brain food rich in healthy fats and memory-enhancing compounds
5. **Avocados** – Loaded with monounsaturated fats and fiber for brain and heart support
6. **Oats & Whole Grains** – Stabilize energy and improve focus by regulating blood sugar
7. **Greek Yogurt** – Rich in probiotics for gut-brain balance and emotional stability
8. **Dark Chocolate (70%+)** – Improves blood flow to the brain and lifts mood naturally
9. **Chickpeas & Lentils** – Plant-based proteins that support neurotransmitter health
10. **Green Tea** – Contains L-theanine and antioxidants for calm focus and long-term brain health

By combining healthy meals with these lifestyle habits, you're supporting not just brain and heart health, but also your mood, energy, and emotional wellness. Every small step counts. The choices you make each day create the foundation for clarity, vitality, and a joyful, independent life.

Let your habits nourish your spirit—one walk, one deep breath, one mindful meal at a time.

Staying Consistent with Healthy Habits

Building healthy habits is one thing. Sticking with them is another. Many people start strong with a new meal plan or fitness routine but struggle to keep going. The secret to long-term success is not perfection. It is **consistency**. The good news is, consistency can be simple when you set yourself up for it.

Start by **making habits easy to follow**. If a recipe feels too long or complicated, you are less likely to make it again. Choose meals you enjoy that take little time and use familiar ingredients. Keep your kitchen stocked with go-to staples. When you reduce daily decisions, you make healthy choices automatic.

Create a **routine that fits your life**. Think about when you feel most energetic. Use that time to prep meals or take a short walk. Morning? Plan breakfast and a stretch. Afternoon? Chop vegetables or set up dinner. Small routines done at the same time each day help build momentum.

Track your habits, not just your goals. Instead of saying, "I want to eat healthy," focus on actions. For example, "I will eat leafy greens three times this week" or "I will drink water before lunch every day." Keep a notebook or calendar and mark off each success. Seeing progress, even in small steps, builds motivation.

Celebrate your wins, no matter how small. Cooked a healthy meal today? That counts. Chose water over soda? That counts too. The brain responds to encouragement. When you notice and appreciate your efforts, you are more likely to keep going.

Be flexible, not rigid. Life happens. You might skip a walk or order takeout once in a while. That is fine. One off day does not erase your progress. The goal is not to be perfect. It is to return to your routine the next day with a positive mindset.

Make it social. Share your healthy habits with someone else. Cook with a friend, walk with a neighbor, or talk about recipes with a family member. You are more likely to stay consistent when someone else is cheering you on.

Set reminders. A note on the fridge, a sticky label near the stove, or an alert on your phone can help nudge you toward good choices. These gentle prompts are like little coaches that keep you on track.

Be patient. Real change takes time. Habits do not form overnight, but they do stick with repetition. Focus on what you can do today. Keep showing up for yourself, one meal, one walk, or one glass of water at a time.

In the end, staying consistent is not about willpower. It is about building a lifestyle that feels natural, rewarding, and sustainable. By creating routines, making it enjoyable, and giving yourself grace, you turn healthy habits into a way of life.

Your body and mind will thank you. Keep going. You are doing something truly good for yourself.

14. GUIDED MEAL PLAN FOR BRAIN HEALTH

Eating for brain health does not have to feel overwhelming. This 21-day MIND diet plan is a senior-friendly, anti inflammatory approach designed to support memory, mood, and long-term cognitive clarity. It blends the best of the Mediterranean and DASH diets to create meals rich in omega 3s, leafy greens, berries, whole grains, nuts, and healthy fats—foods scientifically shown to protect against Alzheimer's and support heart health.

Each day includes breakfast, lunch, dinner, and a snack. Meals are simple, low sodium, and easy to prepare, helping you stay consistent without stress.

Week 1: Getting Started

This week focuses on familiar, brain boosting foods. Keep it simple and repeat your favorites.

Day 1 Example:

- Breakfast: Oatmeal with blueberries and walnuts
- Lunch: Spinach salad with grilled chicken and olive oil
- Snack: Apple slices with almond butter
- Dinner: Baked salmon, brown rice, steamed broccoli

Goals:

- Eat leafy greens daily
- Add one serving of berries
- Use olive oil instead of butter

Week 2: Add Variety

Now it's time to expand your meals with new grains and vegetables.

Sample Meals:

- Quinoa and banana breakfast bowl
- Hummus wrap with carrots and cucumber
- Grilled trout with roasted beets and kale

Tips:

- Try whole grains like quinoa, barley, or farro
- Include two servings of fish this week
- Add lentils or beans for plant-based protein

Week 3: Build Momentum

This week introduces global flavors and encourages more creativity.

Try:

- Mediterranean chickpea salad
- Lentil soup with turmeric
- Dark chocolate with almonds as a snack

Focus:

- Go meatless for two days
- Drink 6–8 glasses of water daily
- Use herbs like garlic, rosemary, and cumin for flavor and wellness

Top 10 Brain & Mood Boosting Foods

Add these to your weekly grocery list:

1. Blueberries
2. Leafy greens
3. Salmon or sardines
4. Walnuts
5. Olive oil
6. Whole grains
7. Chickpeas and lentils
8. Avocados
9. Dark chocolate (70%+)
10. Greek yogurt

Daily Meal Template

- 1–2 servings leafy greens
- 1 serving berries
- Whole grains twice
- Olive oil as main fat
- Nuts, seeds, or legumes
- Drink water throughout the day

Weekly:

- 2+ fish meals
- 4+ meatless meals

- Limit red meat
- Avoid fried foods and sweets

Final Encouragement

You are creating a lifestyle, not just following a diet. Each brain food supports your vitality, mood, and memory. The MIND diet is simple, delicious, and backed by science. Whether you're cooking for one or sharing meals with family, you're taking powerful steps toward healthy aging, cognitive clarity, and overall wellness.

Stick with it. The results will speak for themselves.

PART 3

BRAIN-BOOSTING BREAKFASTS

15: LEAFY GREEN OMELETS & EGG DISHES

Spinach & Feta Omelet

Prep Time: 10 minutes

Serves: 1

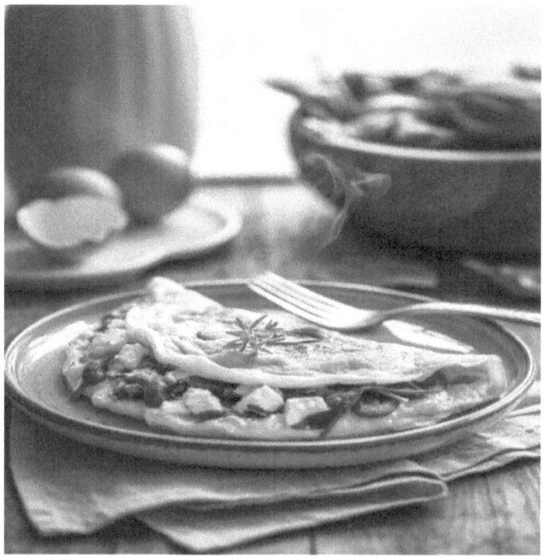

INGREDIENTS:

- 2 eggs
- 1/2 cup fresh spinach, chopped
- 2 tbsp feta cheese, crumbled
- 1 tbsp milk or plant milk
- 1 tsp olive oil
- Salt and pepper to taste

INSTRUCTIONS:

1. Whisk the eggs, milk, salt, and pepper in a bowl until well combined.
2. Heat olive oil in a nonstick skillet over medium heat.
3. Add spinach and sauté for 1 minute until slightly wilted.
4. Pour egg mixture over the spinach and cook undisturbed for 1–2 minutes.

5. Sprinkle feta over one side, fold the omelet, and cook for another minute.
6. Slide onto a plate and serve hot.

Nutrition:

Calories: 220 | **Protein:** 14g | **Fat:** 17g | **Carbohydrates:** 3g | **Fiber:** 1g

Kale & Mushroom Egg Scramble

Prep Time: 12 minutes

Serves: 2

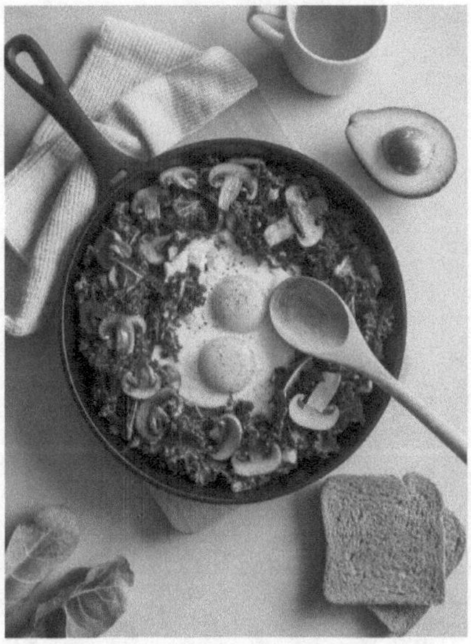

INGREDIENTS:

- 4 eggs
- 1 cup chopped kale
- 1/2 cup sliced mushrooms
- 1/4 cup diced onion
- 1 tbsp olive oil
- Salt and pepper to taste

INSTRUCTIONS:

1. Heat olive oil in a skillet over medium heat.
2. Add onion and mushrooms, and sauté for 3 minutes.
3. Stir in kale and cook until wilted, about 2 minutes.
4. Beat the eggs in a bowl, season, and pour into the pan.

5. Gently scramble the eggs until just set, about 3–4 minutes.
6. Serve warm with a side of whole-grain toast if desired.

Nutrition:

Calories: 180 | **Protein:** 13g | **Fat:** 14g | **Carbohydrates:** 5g | **Fiber:** 2g

Swiss Chard & Goat Cheese Mini Frittatas

Prep Time: 15 minutes

Serves: 4 (makes 8 mini frittatas)

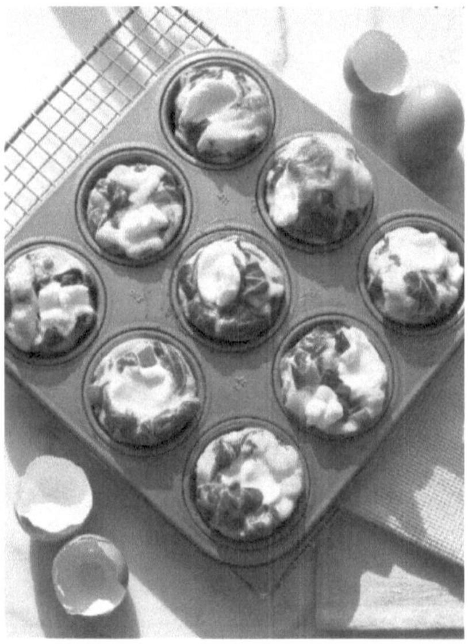

INGREDIENTS:

- 6 eggs
- 1 cup Swiss chard, finely chopped
- 1/3 cup goat cheese, crumbled
- 1/4 cup diced red bell pepper
- 1/4 cup milk or milk alternative
- 1 tsp olive oil
- Salt and pepper to taste

INSTRUCTIONS:

1. Preheat oven to 375°F.
2. Lightly oil a muffin tin or use silicone liners.
3. Sauté chard and bell pepper in olive oil until tender, about 3 minutes.

4. Whisk eggs, milk, salt, and pepper in a large bowl.
5. Stir in the chard mixture and divide evenly among muffin cups.
6. Top each with a bit of goat cheese.
7. Bake for 12–15 minutes until puffed and set.
8. Let cool slightly before serving.

Nutrition:

Calories: 120 (per frittata) | **Protein:** 8g | **Fat:** 9g | **Carbohydrates:** 2g | **Fiber:** 1g |

Arugula & Avocado Egg Toast

Prep Time: 10 minutes

Serves: 1

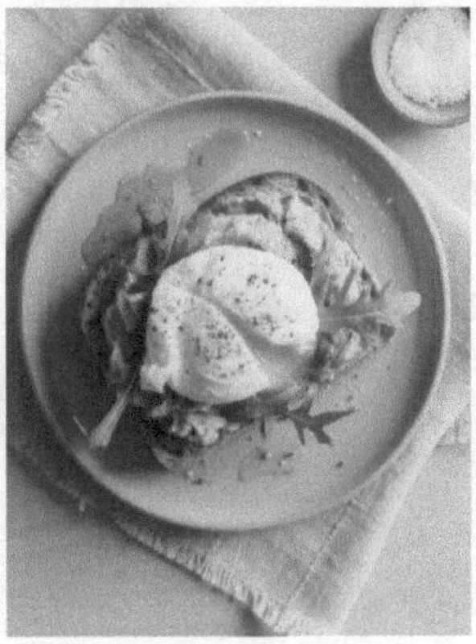

INGREDIENTS:

- 1 slice whole-grain bread, toasted
- 1 egg
- 1/4 avocado, mashed
- 1/4 cup fresh arugula
- 1/2 tsp olive oil
- Salt and pepper to taste

INSTRUCTIONS:

1. Fry or poach the egg to your liking.
2. Spread mashed avocado on the toast.
3. Layer with arugula, then place the cooked egg on top.
4. Drizzle with olive oil and season to taste.

5. Serve immediately for best texture.

Nutrition:

Calories: 260 | **Protein:** 10g | **Fat:** 18g | **Carbohydrates:** 16g | **Fiber:** 5g

Collard Green & Sweet Potato Egg Bake

Prep Time: 20 minutes

Serves: 4

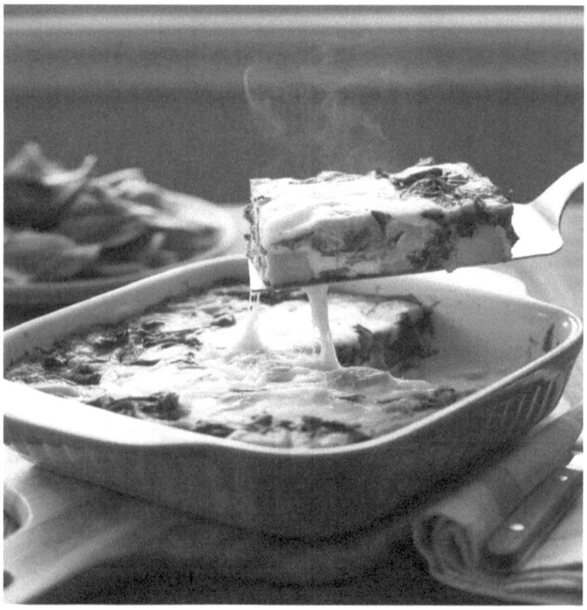

INGREDIENTS:

- 6 eggs
- 1 cup cooked, diced sweet potato
- 1 cup collard greens, chopped
- 1/4 cup diced onion
- 1/4 cup shredded mozzarella or plant-based cheese
- 1/4 cup milk or milk substitute
- 1 tsp olive oil
- Salt and pepper to taste

INSTRUCTIONS:

1. Preheat oven to 375°F.
2. Lightly grease an 8x8 baking dish.

3. Sauté onions and collard greens in olive oil until soft, about 4 minutes.
4. Whisk eggs, milk, salt, and pepper in a large bowl.
5. Stir in sweet potato, collards, onion, and cheese.
6. Pour into baking dish and bake for 20–25 minutes until the center is set.
7. Let cool for 5 minutes before slicing and serving.

Nutrition:

Calories: 210 | **Protein:** 12g | **Fat:** 14g | **Carbohydrates:** 10g | **Fiber:** 2g

16: WHOLE-GRAIN CEREALS & PORRIDGES

Blueberry Walnut Oatmeal

Prep Time: 10 minutes

Serves: 1

INGREDIENTS:

- 1/2 cup rolled oats
- 1 cup water or milk
- 1/4 cup fresh or frozen blueberries
- 1 tbsp chopped walnuts
- 1/2 tsp cinnamon
- Honey or maple syrup to taste (optional)

INSTRUCTIONS:

1. In a small saucepan, bring water or milk to a boil.
2. Stir in oats and reduce heat to simmer.
3. Cook for 5 minutes, stirring occasionally.
4. Stir in blueberries and cinnamon during the last minute.
5. Top with walnuts and a drizzle of honey or syrup if desired.

Nutrition:

Calories: 280 | **Protein:** 6g | **Fat:** 10g | **Carbohydrates:** 42g | **Fiber:** 6g

Quinoa Banana Breakfast Bowl

Prep Time: 15 minutes

Serves: 2

INGREDIENTS:

- 1/2 cup quinoa, rinsed
- 1 cup water or milk
- 1 banana, sliced
- 1 tbsp ground flaxseed
- 1/2 tsp vanilla extract
- 1/2 tsp cinnamon

- 1 tbsp chopped almonds

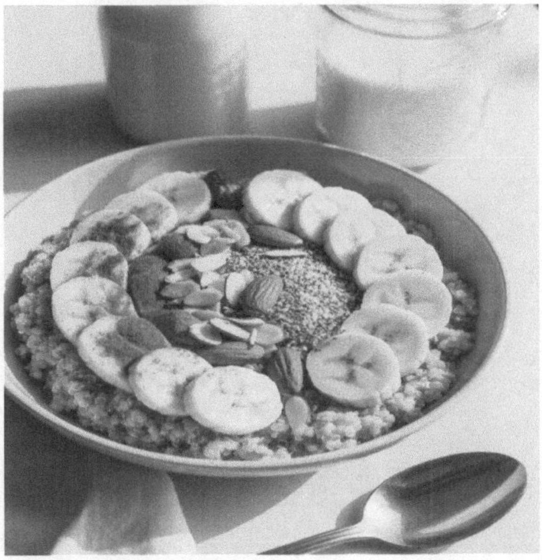

INSTRUCTIONS:

1. In a saucepan, bring quinoa and water or milk to a boil.
2. Reduce heat and simmer for 12–15 minutes until liquid is absorbed.
3. Stir in vanilla, cinnamon, and flaxseed.
4. Divide into bowls and top with banana slices and almonds.

Nutrition:

Calories: 310 | **Protein:** 9g | **Fat:** 9g | **Carbohydrates:** 47g | **Fiber:** 5g

Barley & Apple Warm Cereal

Prep Time: 20 minutes

Serves: 2

INGREDIENTS:

- 1/2 cup pearl barley
- 1 1/2 cups water
- 1 apple, diced
- 1/2 tsp cinnamon
- 1 tbsp raisins
- 1 tsp olive oil or butter
- Pinch of salt

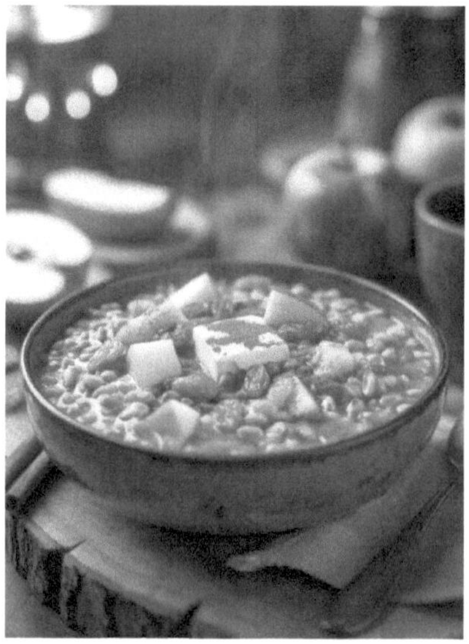

INSTRUCTIONS:

1. Bring water and barley to a boil in a small pot.
2. Reduce heat and simmer uncovered for 15 minutes.
3. Add diced apple, cinnamon, raisins, and salt.
4. Cook for 5 more minutes or until barley is tender.
5. Stir in olive oil or butter and serve warm.

Nutrition:

Calories: 290 | **Protein:** 6g | **Fat:** 5g | **Carbohydrates:** 54g | **Fiber:** 7g | **Vitamin C:** Moderate | **Iron:** Moderate

Savory Oatmeal with Spinach & Egg

Prep Time: 15 minutes

Serves: 1

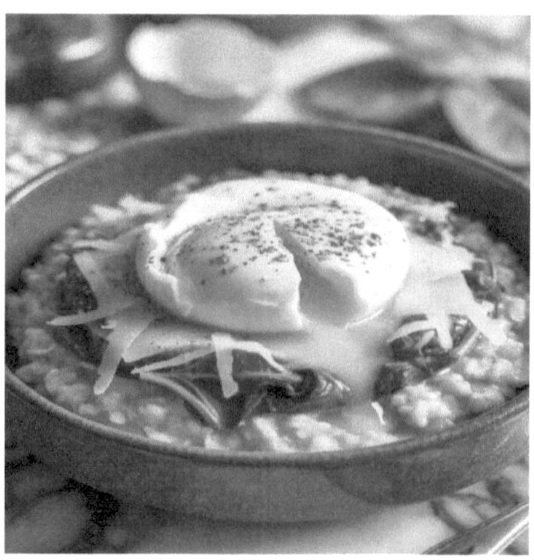

INGREDIENTS:

- 1/2 cup rolled oats
- 1 cup water
- 1/2 cup spinach, chopped
- 1 egg
- 1 tbsp shredded cheese (optional)
- Salt and pepper to taste
- 1 tsp olive oil

INSTRUCTIONS:

1. In a pot, cook oats in water for 5–7 minutes until soft.
2. Stir in spinach and season with salt and pepper.
3. In a separate pan, fry or poach the egg in olive oil.
4. Pour oatmeal into a bowl, top with the egg and cheese if using.
5. Serve warm as a filling, savory breakfast.

Nutrition:

Calories: 310 | **Protein:** 14g | **Fat:** 15g | **Carbohydrates:** 30g | **Fiber:** 4g

Multigrain Chia Porridge

Prep Time: 10 minutes (+overnight soak)

Serves: 2

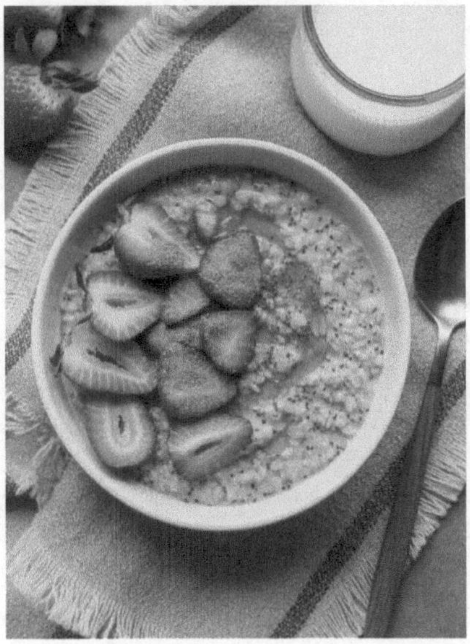

INGREDIENTS:

- 1/2 cup steel-cut oats
- 2 tbsp chia seeds
- 2 tbsp millet or amaranth
- 1 1/2 cups water or milk
- 1 tbsp maple syrup
- 1/4 tsp cinnamon
- 1/4 cup chopped strawberries or berries of choice

INSTRUCTIONS:

1. Combine oats, chia seeds, and millet with water or milk in a bowl.
2. Cover and refrigerate overnight.
3. In the morning, transfer to a saucepan and cook over medium heat for 7–10 minutes, stirring often.
4. Add maple syrup and cinnamon.
5. Top with berries before serving.

Nutrition:

Calories: 270 | **Protein:** 8g | **Fat:** 9g | **Carbohydrates:** 37g | **Fiber:** 7g

17: BERRY-BOOSTED SMOOTHIES

Blueberry Almond Brain Smoothie

Prep Time: 5 minutes

Serves: 1

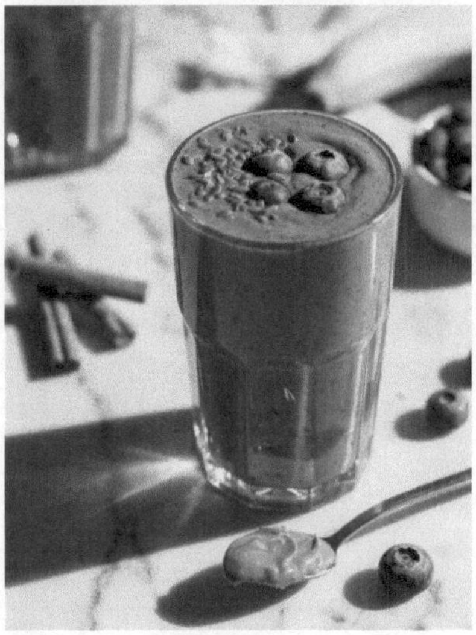

INGREDIENTS:

- 1/2 cup frozen blueberries
- 1/2 banana
- 1 tbsp almond butter
- 1/2 cup unsweetened almond milk
- 1 tbsp ground flaxseed
- 1/4 tsp cinnamon

INSTRUCTIONS:

1. Add all ingredients to a blender.
2. Blend until smooth.
3. Serve immediately for best texture and flavor.

Nutrition:

Calories: 220 | **Protein:** 5g | **Fat:** 12g | **Carbohydrates:** 25g | **Fiber:** 6g | **Omega-3s:** Moderate | **Antioxidants:** High

Strawberry Spinach Power Smoothie

Prep Time: 5 minutes

Serves: 1

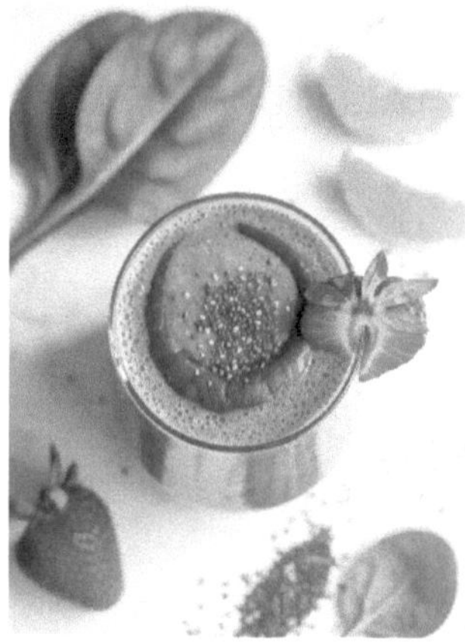

INGREDIENTS:

- 3/4 cup frozen strawberries
- 1/2 cup fresh spinach
- 1/2 cup unsweetened oat milk
- 1/2 orange, peeled and sectioned
- 1 tbsp chia seeds

INSTRUCTIONS:

1. Place all ingredients into a blender.
2. Blend on high speed until creamy.
3. Pour into a glass and enjoy immediately.

Nutrition:

Calories: 180 | **Protein:** 4g | **Fat:** 6g | **Carbohydrates:** 29g | **Fiber:** 7g

Blackberry Walnut Omega Smoothie

Prep Time: 5 minutes

Serves: 1

INGREDIENTS:

- 1/2 cup blackberries
- 1/2 banana
- 1 tbsp chopped walnuts

- 1/2 cup low-fat Greek yogurt
- 1/2 cup water or milk
- 1 tsp honey (optional)

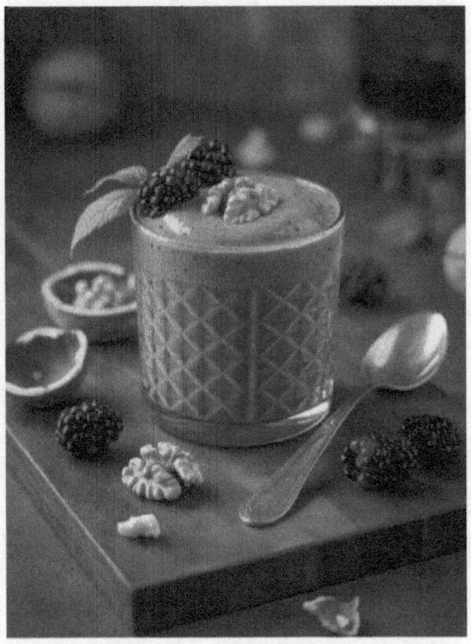

INSTRUCTIONS:

1. Combine blackberries, banana, yogurt, walnuts, and liquid in a blender.
2. Blend until smooth.
3. Add honey for sweetness if desired.

Nutrition:

Calories: 230 | **Protein:** 9g | **Fat:** 10g | **Carbohydrates:** 26g | **Fiber:** 5g

Raspberry Cocoa Memory Smoothie

Prep Time: 5 minutes

Serves: 1

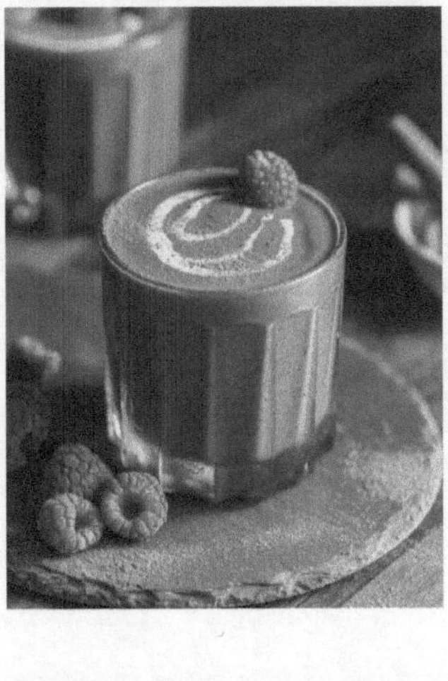

INGREDIENTS:

- 1/2 cup frozen raspberries
- 1/2 cup unsweetened almond milk
- 1/2 frozen banana
- 1 tbsp unsweetened cocoa powder
- 1 tbsp ground flaxseed

INSTRUCTIONS:

1. Add all ingredients to a blender.
2. Blend until thick and smooth.
3. Serve chilled with a sprinkle of cinnamon if desired.

Nutrition:

Calories: 200 | **Protein:** 4g | **Fat:** 9g | **Carbohydrates:** 28g | **Fiber:** 8g

Mixed Berry Green Boost Smoothie

Prep Time: 5 minutes

Serves: 1

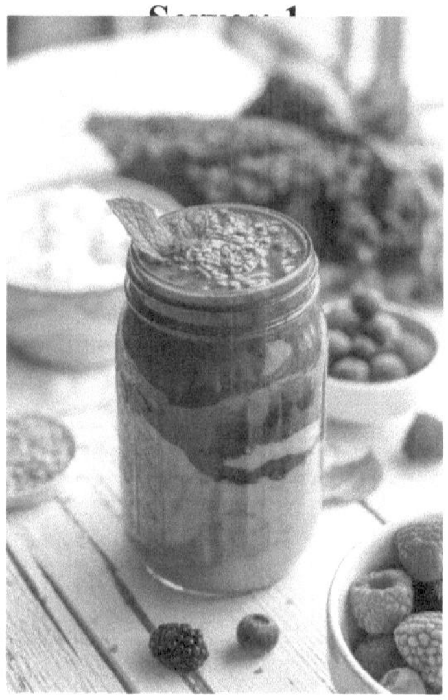

INGREDIENTS:

- 1/2 cup mixed frozen berries (blueberries, strawberries, blackberries)
- 1/2 cup kale or spinach
- 1/2 cup plain Greek yogurt
- 1/2 cup water or milk of choice
- 1 tbsp hemp seeds

INSTRUCTIONS:

1. Place all ingredients in a blender.
2. Blend until smooth and creamy.
3. Pour into a glass and drink immediately.

Nutrition:

Calories: 210 | **Protein:** 10g | **Fat:** 8g | **Carbohydrates:** 23g | **Fiber:** 6g

18. SIMPLE TOASTS & SPREADS WITH HEALTHY FATS

Avocado & Olive Oil Toast

Prep Time: 5 minutes

Serves: 1

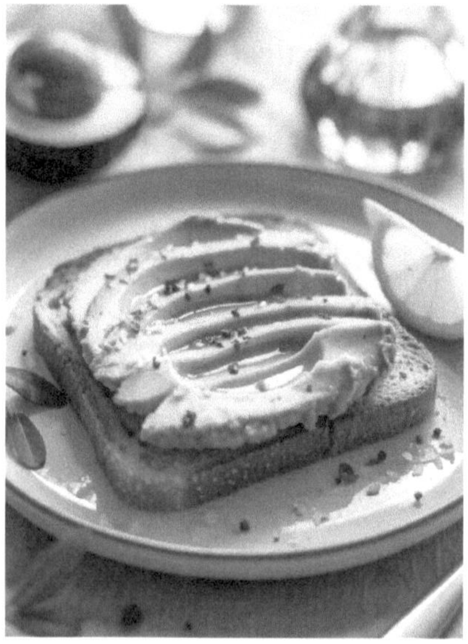

INGREDIENTS:

- 1 slice whole-grain bread, toasted
- 1/2 avocado, mashed
- 1/2 tsp extra virgin olive oil
- Salt and pepper to taste
- Optional: chili flakes or lemon juice

INSTRUCTIONS:

1. Mash the avocado in a small bowl.
2. Spread it over the toasted bread.
3. Drizzle with olive oil and season with salt, pepper, and optional toppings.
4. Serve immediately.

Nutrition:

Calories: 250 | **Protein:** 6g | **Fat:** 18g | **Carbohydrates:** 20g | **Fiber:** 7g

Nut Butter & Blueberry Toast

Prep Time: 5 minutes

Serves: 1

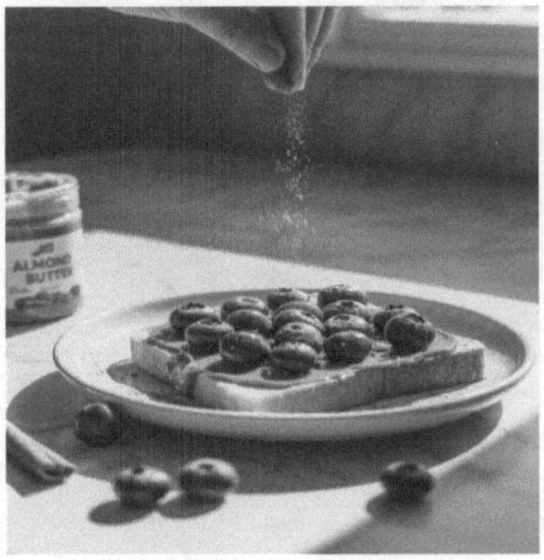

INGREDIENTS:

- 1 slice whole-grain bread, toasted
- 1 tbsp natural almond or peanut butter
- 1/4 cup fresh blueberries
- Dash of cinnamon

INSTRUCTIONS:

1. Spread the nut butter on the toast.
2. Top with blueberries and sprinkle with cinnamon.
3. Serve fresh for best texture.

Nutrition:

Calories: 240 | **Protein:** 7g | **Fat:** 14g | **Carbohydrates:** 22g | **Fiber:** 5g | **Vitamin E:** High | **Antioxidants:** High

Hummus & Cucumber Rye Toast

Prep Time: 5 minutes

Serves: 1

INGREDIENTS:

- 1 slice rye or whole-grain bread, toasted
- 2 tbsp hummus
- 1/4 cup thinly sliced cucumber
- 1 tsp lemon juice

- Fresh dill or parsley (optional)

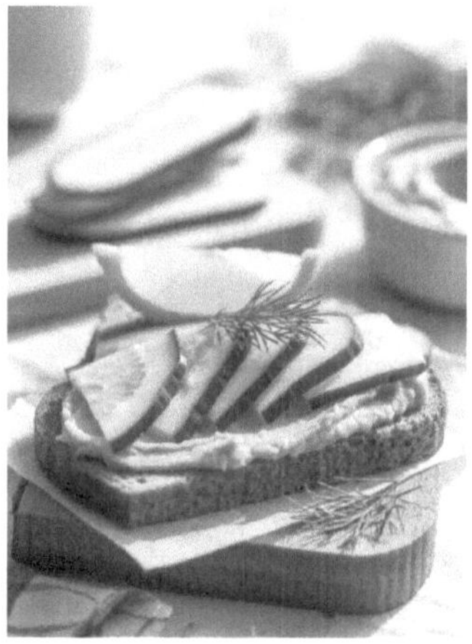

INSTRUCTIONS:

1. Spread hummus on the toast.
2. Arrange cucumber slices on top.
3. Drizzle with lemon juice and garnish with fresh herbs.
4. Enjoy immediately.

Nutrition:

Calories: 190 | **Protein:** 6g | **Fat:** 9g | **Carbohydrates:** 20g | **Fiber:** 4g | **Folate:** Moderate | **Plant Protein:** Moderate

Ricotta & Walnut Fig Toast

Prep Time: 7 minutes

Serves: 1

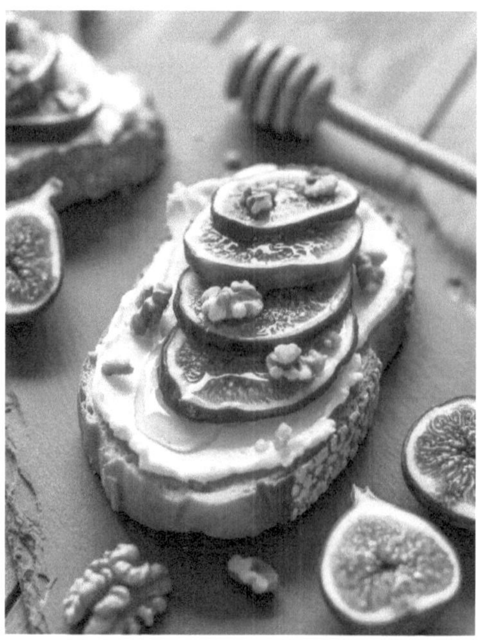

INGREDIENTS:

- 1 slice whole-grain or sourdough bread, toasted
- 2 tbsp ricotta cheese
- 1 dried fig, sliced thin
- 1 tsp chopped walnuts
- Optional: drizzle of honey

INSTRUCTIONS:

1. Spread ricotta over warm toast.
2. Top with fig slices and walnuts.
3. Add a drizzle of honey if desired.
4. Serve warm.

Nutrition:

Calories: 230 | **Protein:** 8g | **Fat:** 10g | **Carbohydrates:** 26g | **Fiber:** 3g |

Avocado & Egg Toast

Prep Time: 10 minutes

Serves: 1

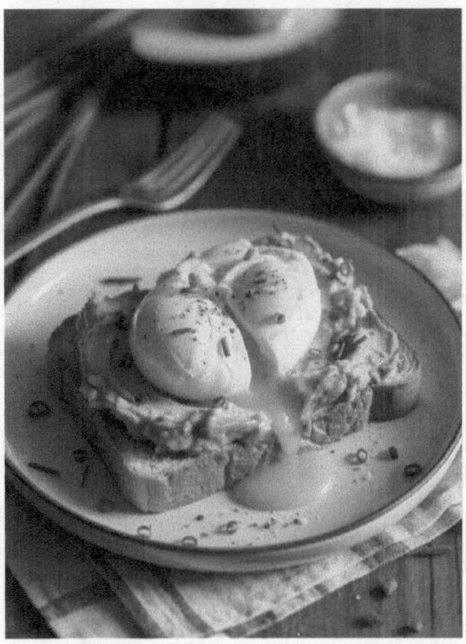

INGREDIENTS:

- 1 slice whole-grain bread, toasted
- 1/4 avocado, mashed
- 1 poached or fried egg

- Salt and black pepper to taste
- Optional: paprika or chopped chives

INSTRUCTIONS:

1. Spread mashed avocado over toast.
2. Top with the cooked egg.
3. Season with salt, pepper, and optional garnish.
4. Serve warm with a side of fruit or greens.

Nutrition:

Calories: 270 | **Protein:** 11g | **Fat:** 18g | **Carbohydrates:** 18g | **Fiber:** 5g

19. BRAINY BREAKFAST BOWLS

Berry Quinoa Yogurt Bowl

Prep Time: 10 minutes

Serves: 1

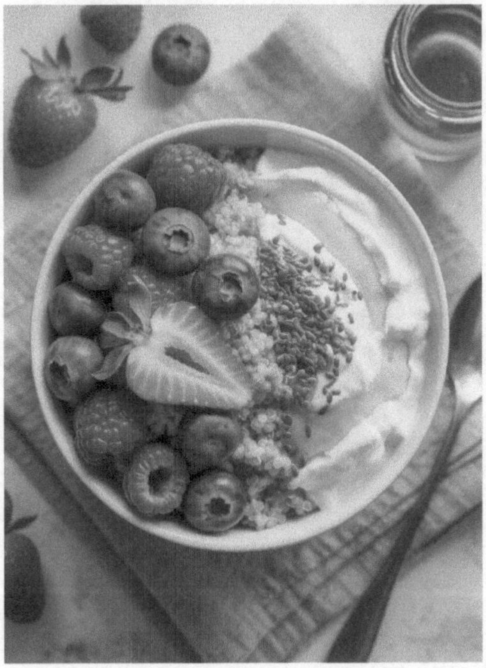

INGREDIENTS:

- 1/2 cup cooked quinoa (cooled)
- 1/2 cup plain Greek yogurt
- 1/4 cup mixed berries (blueberries, raspberries, strawberries)
- 1 tbsp ground flaxseed
- 1 tsp honey (optional)

INSTRUCTIONS:

1. In a bowl, combine the quinoa and yogurt.
2. Top with berries and flaxseed.
3. Drizzle with honey if desired.
4. Serve chilled or at room temperature.

Nutrition:

Calories: 280 | **Protein:** 15g | **Fat:** 8g | **Carbohydrates:** 33g | **Fiber:** 5g

Savory Sweet Potato & Egg Bowl

Prep Time: 15 minutes

Serves: 1

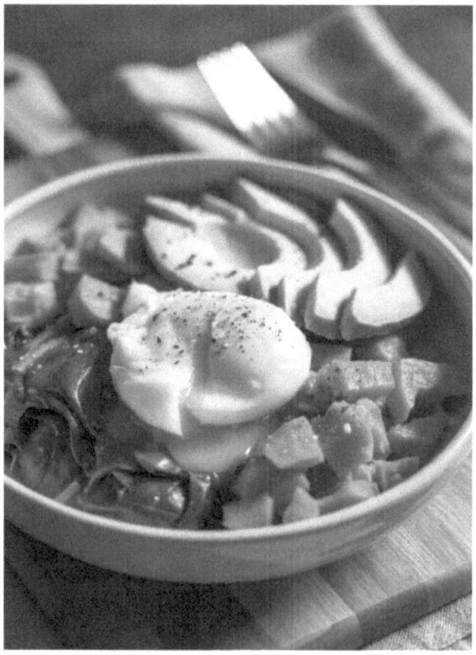

INGREDIENTS:

- 1/2 cup cooked sweet potato, diced
- 1 egg, poached or fried
- 1/4 avocado, sliced
- 1/2 cup sautéed spinach
- Salt and pepper to taste

INSTRUCTIONS:

1. Arrange sweet potato, avocado, and spinach in a bowl.
2. Top with the cooked egg.
3. Season with salt and pepper.
4. Serve warm.

Nutrition:

Calories: 310 | **Protein:** 11g | **Fat:** 17g | **Carbohydrates:** 28g | **Fiber:** 6g | **Vitamin A:** High | **Healthy Fats:** High

Chia & Oat Power Bowl

Prep Time: 5 minutes + overnight soak

Serves: 1

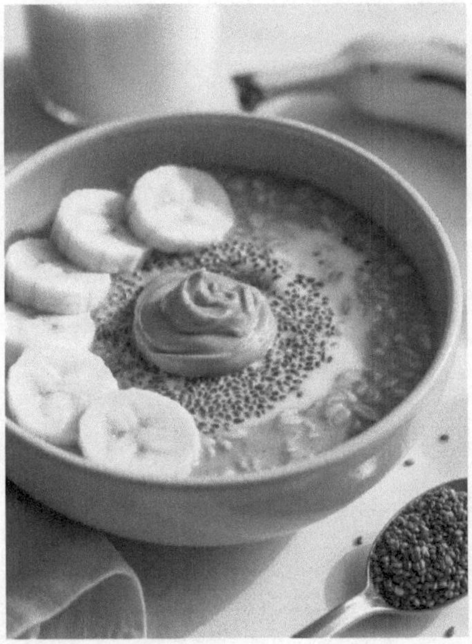

INGREDIENTS:

- 1/4 cup rolled oats
- 1 tbsp chia seeds
- 1/2 cup milk or plant milk
- 1/2 banana, sliced
- 1 tbsp peanut butter

INSTRUCTIONS:

1. In a jar or bowl, combine oats, chia seeds, and milk.
2. Stir well and refrigerate overnight.
3. In the morning, top with banana slices and peanut butter.
4. Serve chilled or bring to room temperature.

Nutrition:

Calories: 300 | **Protein:** 9g | **Fat:** 13g | **Carbohydrates:** 35g | **Fiber:** 8g | **Magnesium:** Moderate | **Plant Protein:** Moderate

Green Veggie Grain Bowl

Prep Time: 10 minutes

Serves: 1

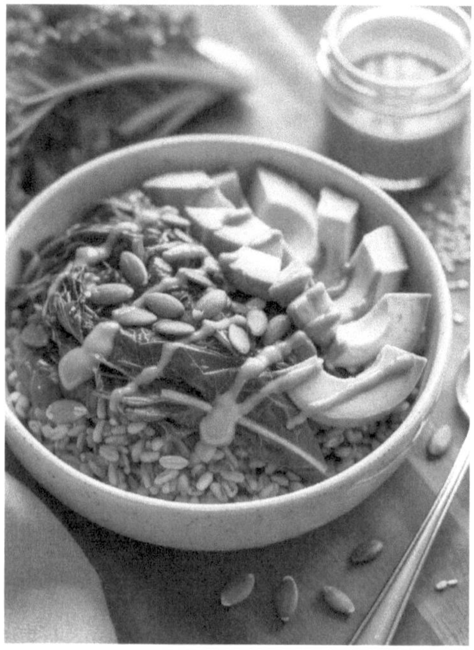

INGREDIENTS:

- 1/2 cup cooked brown rice or farro
- 1/2 cup sautéed kale or collard greens
- 1/4 avocado, diced
- 1 tbsp pumpkin seeds
- 1 tbsp tahini or olive oil

INSTRUCTIONS:

1. Place cooked grain in a bowl as the base.
2. Layer with greens and avocado.
3. Sprinkle with pumpkin seeds and drizzle with tahini or olive oil.
4. Serve warm or at room temperature.

Nutrition:

Calories: 330 | **Protein:** 9g | **Fat:** 18g | **Carbohydrates:** 32g | **Fiber:** 6g | **Zinc:** Moderate | **Vitamin K:** High

Cottage Cheese & Berry Brain Bowl

Prep Time: 5 minutes

Serves: 1

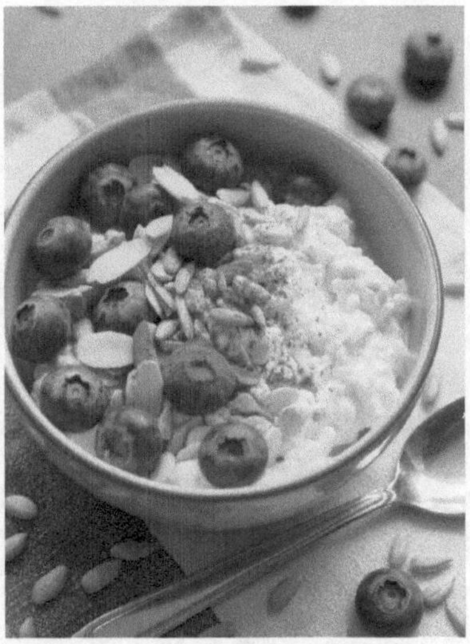

INGREDIENTS:

- 1/2 cup low-fat cottage cheese
- 1/4 cup blueberries
- 1 tbsp sliced almonds
- 1 tbsp sunflower seeds
- Dash of cinnamon

INSTRUCTIONS:

1. Spoon cottage cheese into a bowl.
2. Top with blueberries, almonds, and sunflower seeds.
3. Sprinkle with cinnamon.
4. Serve immediately.

Nutrition:

Calories: 240 | **Protein:** 16g | **Fat:** 10g | **Carbohydrates:** 15g | **Fiber:** 3g

20. ON-THE-GO SENIOR-FRIENDLY MORNING MEALS

Oatmeal Muffin Cups

Prep Time: 10 minutes + 20 minutes baking

Serves: 6 muffins

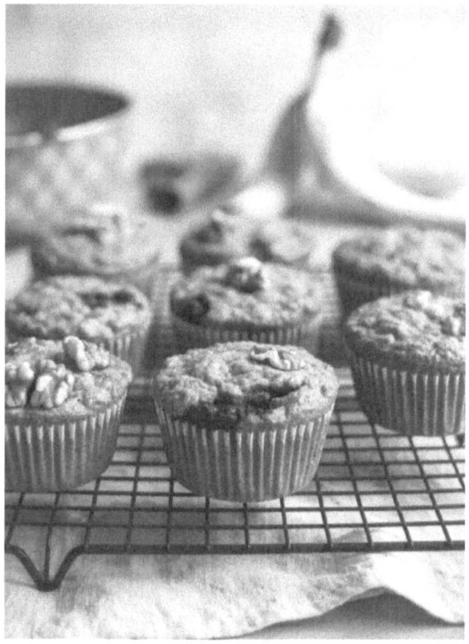

INGREDIENTS:

- 1 cup rolled oats
- 1/2 cup mashed banana
- 1/2 cup unsweetened applesauce
- 1/2 tsp cinnamon
- 1/4 cup chopped walnuts
- 1/4 cup blueberries
- 1 egg

INSTRUCTIONS:

1. Preheat oven to 350°F and grease a muffin tin.
2. In a bowl, mix all ingredients until combined.
3. Spoon mixture evenly into 6 muffin cups.
4. Bake for 20 minutes or until golden and set.
5. Let cool and store in the fridge for up to 5 days.

Nutrition:

Calories: 140 | **Protein:** 4g | **Fat:** 5g | **Carbohydrates:** 21g | **Fiber:** 3g | **Portable:** Yes | **Brain Fuel:** Moderate

Avocado Egg Wrap

Prep Time: 10 minutes

Serves: 1

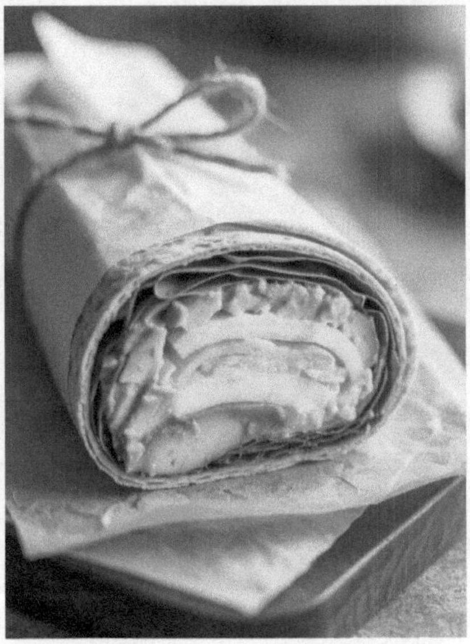

INGREDIENTS:

- 1 whole wheat tortilla
- 1 hard-boiled egg, sliced
- 1/4 avocado, mashed
- 1/4 cup baby spinach
- Salt and pepper to taste

INSTRUCTIONS:

1. Spread mashed avocado on the tortilla.
2. Layer with spinach and egg slices.
3. Season to taste and roll tightly.
4. Wrap in foil or parchment if taking to-go.

Nutrition:

Calories: 260 | **Protein:** 11g | **Fat:** 15g | **Carbohydrates:** 21g | **Fiber:** 5g

Nut Butter & Banana Sandwich Thin

Prep Time: 3 minutes

Serves: 1

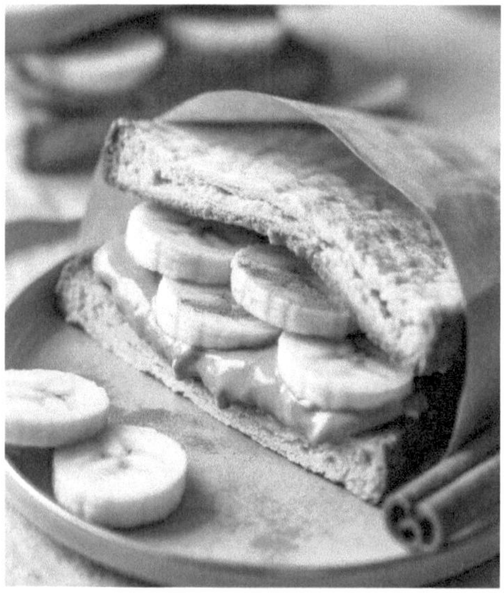

INGREDIENTS:

- 1 whole grain sandwich thin, split
- 1 tbsp natural peanut or almond butter
- 1/2 banana, sliced
- Dash of cinnamon

INSTRUCTIONS:

1. Spread nut butter on one half of the sandwich thin.
2. Top with banana slices and sprinkle with cinnamon.
3. Close with the other half and enjoy or wrap to take with you.

Nutrition:

Calories: 230 | **Protein:** 7g | **Fat:** 11g | **Carbohydrates:** 26g | **Fiber:** 4g

Greek Yogurt Parfait Jar

Prep Time: 5 minutes

Serves: 1

INGREDIENTS:

- 1/2 cup plain Greek yogurt
- 1/4 cup mixed berries

- 1 tbsp chopped walnuts or granola
- 1 tsp honey (optional)

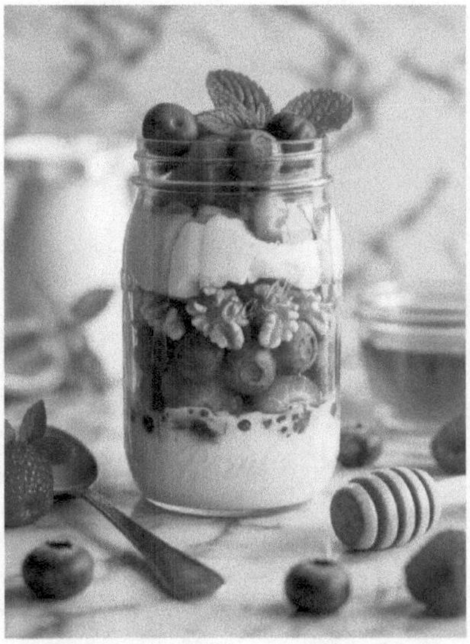

INSTRUCTIONS:

1. In a jar or container, layer yogurt, berries, and nuts or granola.
2. Drizzle with honey if desired.
3. Seal and refrigerate or take on the go.

Nutrition:

Calories: 200 | **Protein:** 12g | **Fat:** 8g | **Carbohydrates:** 16g | **Fiber:** 2g

Chia Pudding To-Go Cup

Prep Time: 5 minutes + 4 hours chill

Serves: 1

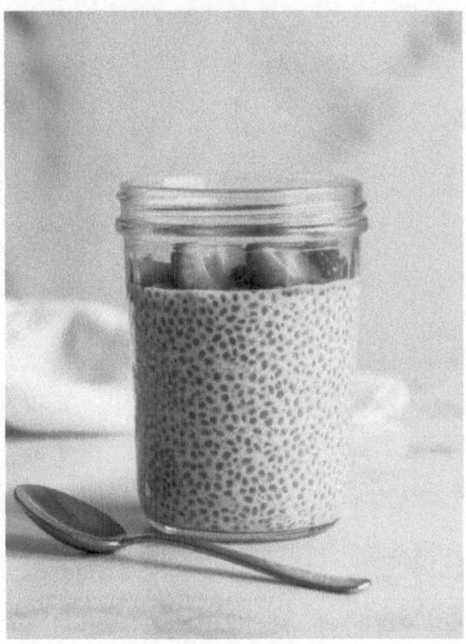

INGREDIENTS:

- 2 tbsp chia seeds
- 1/2 cup milk or plant-based milk
- 1/2 tsp vanilla extract
- 1/4 cup berries or sliced fruit

INSTRUCTIONS:

1. Stir chia seeds, milk, and vanilla in a jar or container.
2. Cover and refrigerate for at least 4 hours or overnight.
3. Top with fruit before serving or pack as is for a grab-and-go option.

Nutrition:

Calories: 180 | **Protein:** 5g | **Fat:** 9g | **Carbohydrates:** 20g | **Fiber:** 6g

PART 4

NOURISHING LUNCHES & DINNERS

21. HEARTY SOUPS & STEWS FOR COGNITIVE CLARITY

Lentil & Spinach Brain Stew

Prep Time: 10 minutes + 25 minutes simmer

Serves: 4

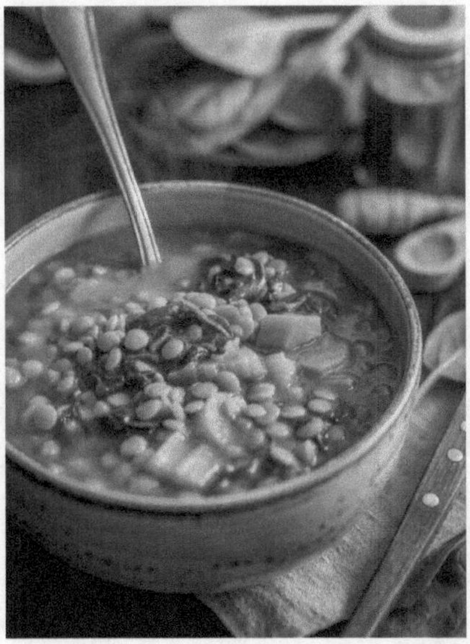

INGREDIENTS:

- 1 cup dried brown or green lentils, rinsed
- 1 tbsp olive oil
- 1/2 onion, diced
- 2 garlic cloves, minced
- 1 carrot, diced
- 1 celery stalk, chopped
- 1/2 tsp turmeric
- 4 cups low-sodium vegetable broth
- 2 cups fresh spinach
- Salt and pepper to taste

INSTRUCTIONS:

1. Heat olive oil in a large pot over medium heat.

2. Add onion, garlic, carrot, and celery. Sauté for 5 minutes.
3. Stir in turmeric and lentils. Add broth and bring to a boil.
4. Reduce heat and simmer uncovered for 25 minutes, or until lentils are soft.
5. Stir in spinach and cook for 2 more minutes.
6. Season with salt and pepper. Serve hot.

Nutrition:

Calories: 260 | **Protein:** 15g | **Fat:** 6g | **Carbohydrates:** 38g | **Fiber:** 10g

Salmon & Sweet Potato Chowder

Prep Time: 15 minutes + 20 minutes simmer

Serves: 3

INGREDIENTS:

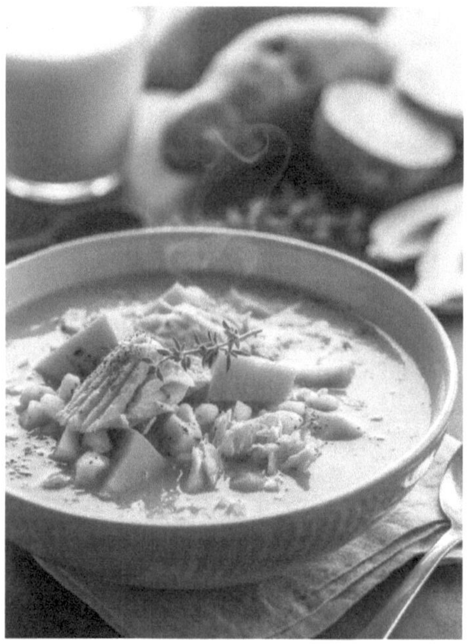

- 1 tbsp olive oil
- 1/2 onion, chopped
- 1 small sweet potato, diced
- 2 cups low-sodium fish or vegetable broth
- 1/2 cup unsweetened almond milk
- 1 cup cooked salmon, flaked
- 1/2 tsp thyme
- Salt and pepper to taste

INSTRUCTIONS:

1. In a pot, heat olive oil and sauté onion for 3–4 minutes.
2. Add sweet potato and thyme. Stir to coat.
3. Pour in broth and bring to a boil.
4. Reduce heat and simmer for 15 minutes, or until potatoes are tender.
5. Stir in almond milk and salmon. Simmer 5 more minutes.
6. Season and serve warm.

Nutrition:

Calories: 310 | **Protein:** 22g | **Fat:** 14g | **Carbohydrates:** 22g | **Fiber:** 4g

White Bean & Kale Garlic Soup

Prep Time: 10 minutes + 20 minutes simmer

Serves: 4

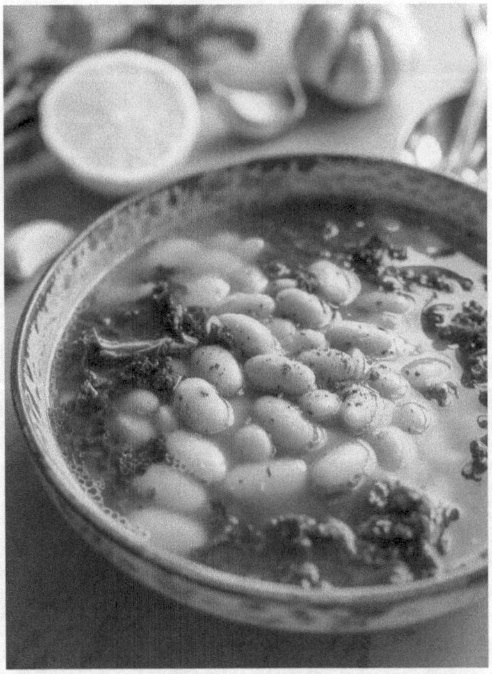

INGREDIENTS:

- 1 tbsp olive oil
- 3 garlic cloves, minced
- 1/2 onion, diced
- 1 can (15 oz) white beans, rinsed
- 3 cups low-sodium vegetable broth

- 2 cups chopped kale
- 1 tsp lemon juice
- Salt and pepper to taste

INSTRUCTIONS:

1. Heat olive oil in a pot and sauté garlic and onion for 4 minutes.
2. Add beans and broth. Bring to a boil.
3. Reduce heat, add kale, and simmer for 15 minutes.
4. Stir in lemon juice, season, and serve.

Nutrition:

Calories: 230 | **Protein:** 10g | **Fat:** 8g | **Carbohydrates:** 30g | **Fiber:** 8g

Mushroom & Barley Mental Boost Soup

Prep Time: 10 minutes + 30 minutes simmer

Serves: 4

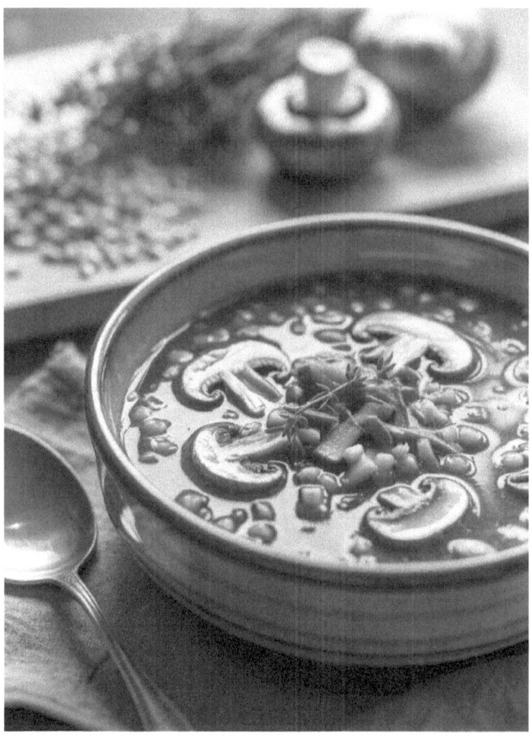

INGREDIENTS:

- 1 tbsp olive oil
- 1/2 onion, chopped
- 2 cups mushrooms, sliced

- 1/2 cup pearl barley
- 4 cups low-sodium vegetable broth
- 1/2 tsp thyme
- Salt and pepper to taste

INSTRUCTIONS:

1. Heat oil in a pot and sauté onion and mushrooms for 5–6 minutes.
2. Stir in barley and thyme.
3. Add broth and bring to a boil.
4. Simmer uncovered for 30 minutes until barley is tender.
5. Season to taste and serve hot.

Nutrition:

Calories: 240 | **Protein:** 7g | **Fat:** 7g | **Carbohydrates:** 38g | **Fiber:** 6g

Tomato Basil Chickpea Stew

Prep Time: 10 minutes + 20 minutes simmer

Serves: 4

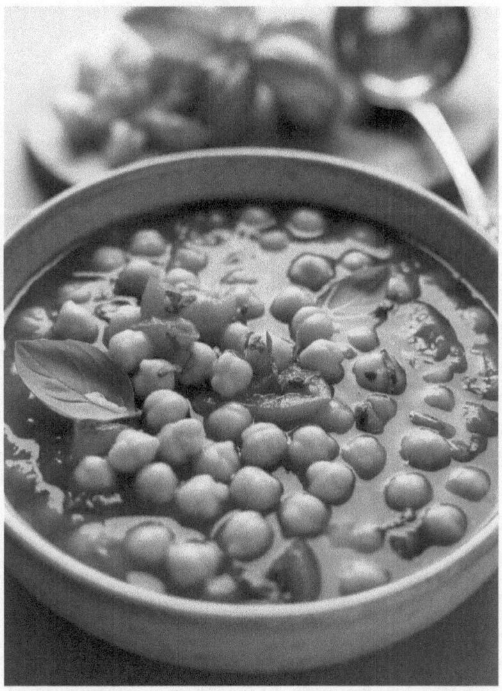

INGREDIENTS:

- 1 tbsp olive oil
- 2 garlic cloves, minced

- 1/2 onion, diced
- 1 can (15 oz) chickpeas, drained
- 1 can (15 oz) diced tomatoes
- 2 cups low-sodium vegetable broth
- 1 tsp dried basil
- Salt and pepper to taste

INSTRUCTIONS:

1. Heat olive oil in a pot over medium heat.
2. Sauté garlic and onion until softened, about 4 minutes.
3. Add chickpeas, tomatoes, broth, and basil. Stir well.
4. Simmer uncovered for 20 minutes.
5. Season to taste and serve warm with optional whole-grain bread.

Nutrition:

Calories: 270 | **Protein:** 12g | **Fat:** 8g | **Carbohydrates:** 34g | **Fiber:** 9g

22. POWER SALADS WITH LEAFY GREENS & NUTS

Walnut Spinach Berry Salad

Prep Time: 10 minutes

Serves: 2

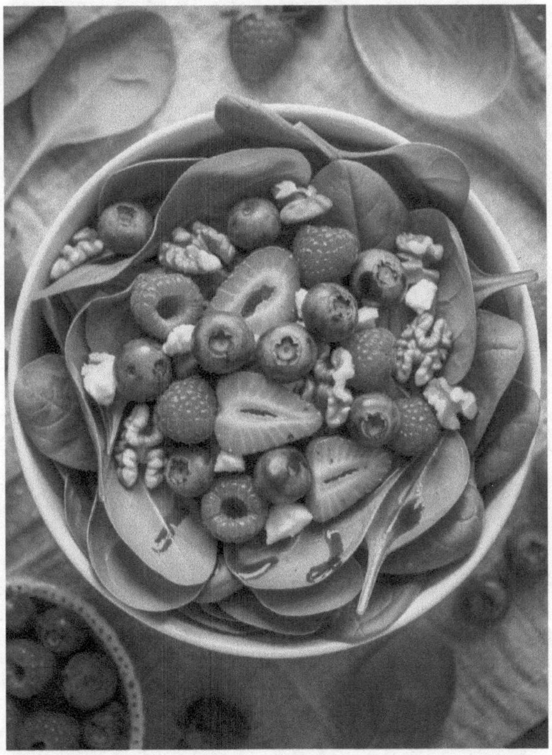

INGREDIENTS:

- 3 cups fresh spinach
- 1/2 cup mixed berries (blueberries, strawberries, raspberries)
- 1/4 cup chopped walnuts
- 2 tbsp crumbled feta (optional)
- 1 tbsp olive oil
- 1 tsp balsamic vinegar

INSTRUCTIONS:

1. In a large bowl, toss together spinach, berries, and walnuts.
2. Add feta if using.
3. Drizzle with olive oil and balsamic vinegar.
4. Toss gently and serve fresh.

Nutrition:

Calories: 210 | **Protein:** 5g | **Fat:** 17g | **Carbohydrates:** 14g | **Fiber:** 4g |

Kale Apple Almond Crunch Salad

Prep Time: 12 minutes

Serves: 2

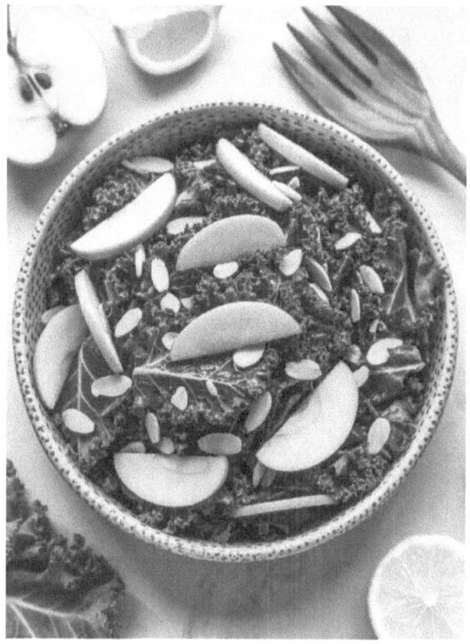

INGREDIENTS:

- 2 cups kale, stems removed and chopped
- 1 small apple, sliced thin
- 1/4 cup sliced almonds
- 1 tbsp olive oil
- 1 tsp lemon juice
- Salt and pepper to taste

INSTRUCTIONS:

1. In a bowl, massage kale with olive oil for 1–2 minutes to soften.
2. Add apple slices and almonds.
3. Drizzle with lemon juice.
4. Season with salt and pepper. Toss and serve.

Nutrition:

Calories: 190 | **Protein:** 4g | **Fat:** 14g | **Carbohydrates:** 15g | **Fiber:** 5g

Arugula Walnut Beet Salad

Prep Time: 10 minutes

Serves: 2

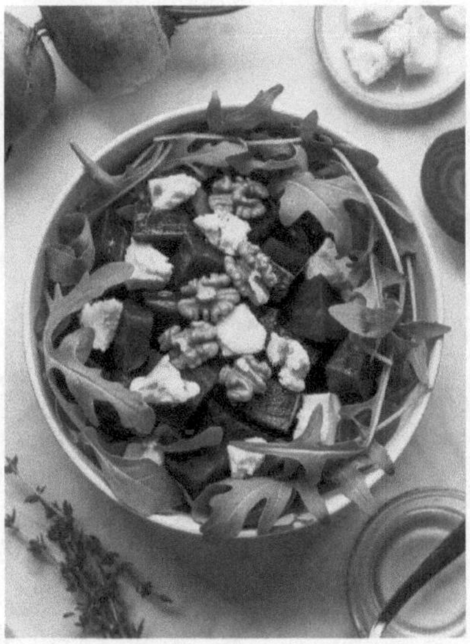

INGREDIENTS:

- 2 cups arugula
- 1/2 cup cooked beets, diced
- 1/4 cup chopped walnuts
- 1 tbsp goat cheese or feta
- 1 tbsp olive oil
- 1 tsp red wine vinegar

INSTRUCTIONS:

1. Combine arugula, beets, and walnuts in a bowl.
2. Add goat cheese on top.
3. Drizzle with olive oil and vinegar.
4. Toss gently and serve chilled or at room temperature.

Nutrition:

Calories: 220 | **Protein:** 6g | **Fat:** 17g | **Carbohydrates:** 13g | **Fiber:** 4g

Chickpea Avocado Romaine Salad

Prep Time: 10 minutes

Serves: 2

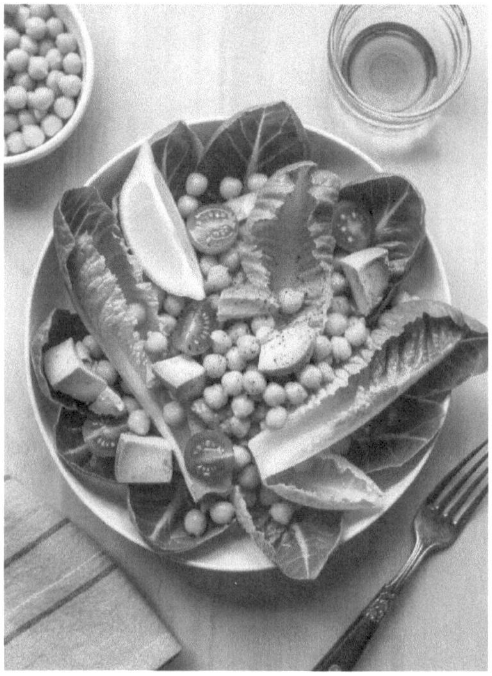

INGREDIENTS:

- 2 cups chopped romaine lettuce
- 1/2 cup canned chickpeas, rinsed
- 1/2 avocado, diced
- 1/4 cup cherry tomatoes, halved
- 1 tbsp olive oil
- 1 tsp lemon juice

INSTRUCTIONS:

1. In a salad bowl, combine romaine, chickpeas, avocado, and tomatoes.
2. Drizzle with olive oil and lemon juice.
3. Toss well and serve immediately.

Nutrition:

Calories: 240 | **Protein:** 7g | **Fat:** 15g | **Carbohydrates:** 20g | **Fiber:** 6g | **Folate:** High | **Healthy Fats:** High

Mixed Greens & Pistachio Citrus Salad

Prep Time: 8 minutes

Serves: 2

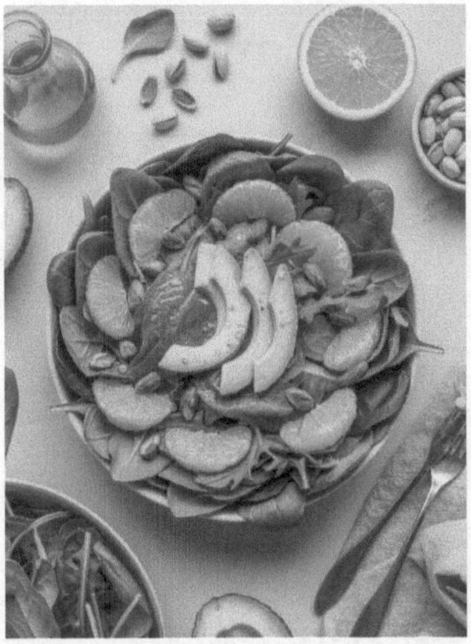

INGREDIENTS:

- 2 cups mixed leafy greens (spinach, arugula, romaine)
- 1/2 orange, segmented
- 1/4 avocado, sliced
- 2 tbsp shelled pistachios
- 1 tbsp olive oil
- 1 tsp apple cider vinegar

INSTRUCTIONS:

1. Place greens in a large bowl.
2. Add orange segments, avocado, and pistachios.
3. Drizzle with olive oil and vinegar.
4. Toss lightly and serve chilled.

Nutrition:

Calories: 210 | **Protein:** 5g | **Fat:** 16g | **Carbohydrates:** 15g | **Fiber:** 5g

23. GRAIN BOWLS WITH OMEGA-3 PROTEINS

Salmon Quinoa Power Bowl

Prep Time: 15 minutes

Serves: 2

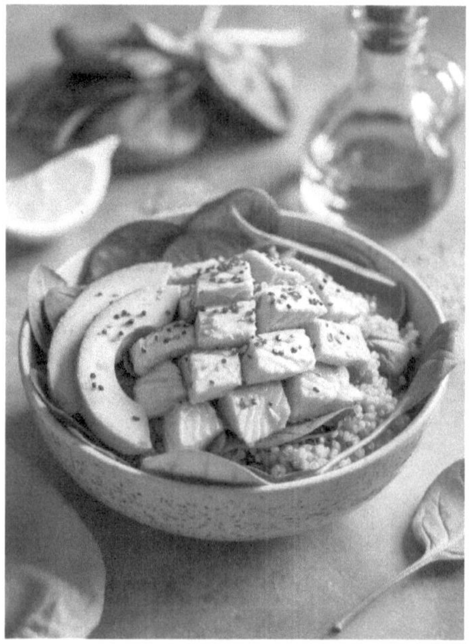

INGREDIENTS:

- 1/2 cup cooked quinoa
- 1/2 cup cooked salmon, flaked
- 1 cup baby spinach
- 1/4 avocado, sliced
- 1 tbsp olive oil
- 1 tsp lemon juice
- Salt and pepper to taste

INSTRUCTIONS:

1. Divide quinoa between two bowls.
2. Top with spinach, salmon, and avocado.
3. Drizzle with olive oil and lemon juice.
4. Season to taste and serve warm or cold.

Nutrition:

Calories: 350 | **Protein:** 22g | **Fat:** 20g | **Carbohydrates:** 18g | **Fiber:** 4g

Sardine Brown Rice Bowl

Prep Time: 10 minutes

Serves: 2

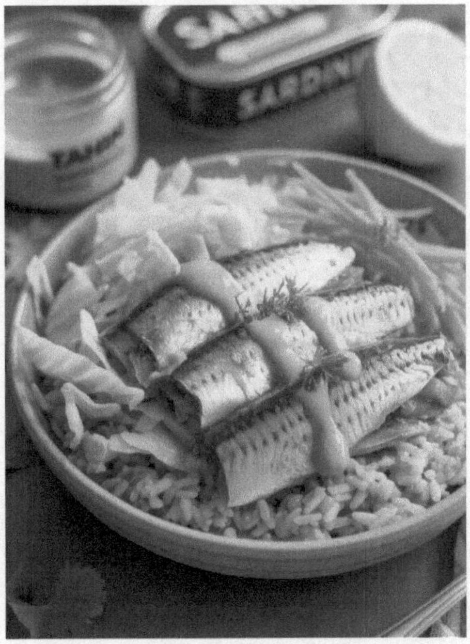

INGREDIENTS:

- 1 cup cooked brown rice
- 1 can sardines in olive oil, drained
- 1/2 cup shredded lettuce or cabbage
- 1/4 cup grated carrot
- 1 tbsp tahini
- 1 tsp lemon juice

INSTRUCTIONS:

1. Layer rice in each bowl.
2. Top with sardines, lettuce, and carrot.
3. Whisk tahini and lemon juice together and drizzle over each bowl.
4. Serve immediately or chill for later.

Nutrition:

Calories: 370 | **Protein:** 21g | **Fat:** 22g | **Carbohydrates:** 24g | **Fiber:** 3g

Walnut Lentil Farro Bowl

Prep Time: 15 minutes

Serves: 2

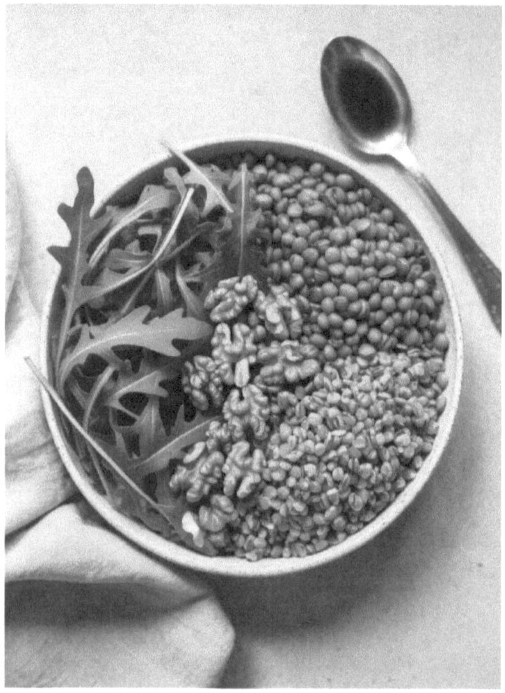

INGREDIENTS:

- 1/2 cup cooked farro
- 1/2 cup cooked lentils
- 1/4 cup chopped walnuts
- 1/2 cup arugula
- 1 tbsp olive oil
- 1 tsp balsamic vinegar

INSTRUCTIONS:

1. Mix farro and lentils and divide between bowls.
2. Add arugula and walnuts on top.
3. Drizzle with olive oil and balsamic vinegar.
4. Toss gently and serve.

Nutrition:

Calories: 320 | **Protein:** 15g | **Fat:** 16g | **Carbohydrates:** 30g | **Fiber:** 6g | **Plant Omega-3s:** High | **Iron:** Moderate

Tuna Millet Veggie Bowl

Prep Time: 15 minutes

Serves: 2

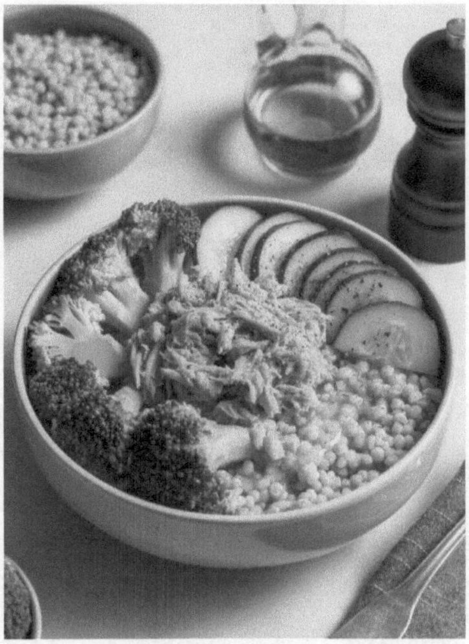

INGREDIENTS:

- 1/2 cup cooked millet
- 1 can tuna in water, drained
- 1/2 cup steamed broccoli
- 1/4 cup sliced cucumber
- 1 tbsp olive oil
- 1 tsp apple cider vinegar
- Black pepper to taste

INSTRUCTIONS:

1. Place millet in the bottom of each bowl.
2. Top with tuna, broccoli, and cucumber.
3. Drizzle with olive oil and vinegar.
4. Sprinkle with black pepper and serve.

Nutrition:

Calories: 330 | **Protein:** 25g | **Fat:** 14g | **Carbohydrates:** 26g | **Fiber:** 5g

Chia-Boosted Barley & Mackerel Bowl

Prep Time: 20 minutes

Serves: 2

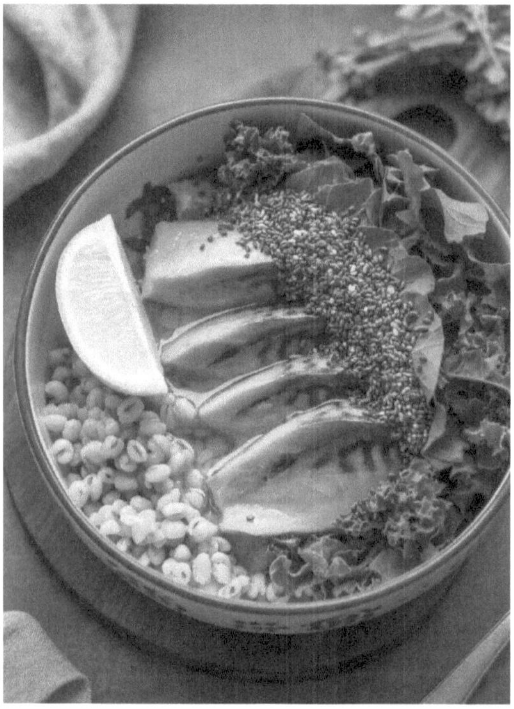

INGREDIENTS:

- 1/2 cup cooked barley
- 1 small can mackerel in olive oil, flaked
- 1/2 cup shredded kale
- 1 tbsp chia seeds
- 1 tbsp olive oil
- 1 tsp lemon juice

INSTRUCTIONS:

1. Layer barley into each bowl.
2. Top with kale, mackerel, and chia seeds.
3. Drizzle with olive oil and lemon juice.
4. Serve immediately or refrigerate.

Nutrition:

Calories: 360 | **Protein:** 20g | **Fat:** 22g | **Carbohydrates:** 22g | **Fiber:** 5g | **Omega-3s:** Very High | **Brain & Heart Support:** Strong

24. ALZHEIMER'S-FIGHTING FISH & POULTRY MEALS

Lemon Herb Baked Salmon

Prep Time: 10 minutes + 15 minutes baking

Serves: 2

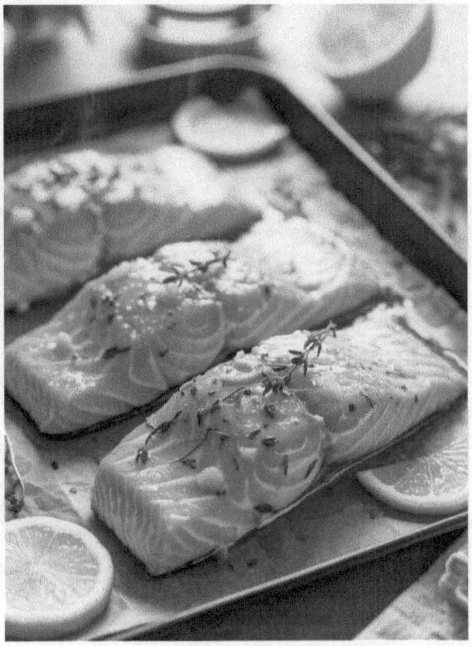

INGREDIENTS:

- 2 salmon fillets (about 4 oz each)
- 1 tbsp olive oil
- 1 tsp lemon zest
- 1 tbsp lemon juice
- 1/2 tsp dried thyme
- Salt and pepper to taste

INSTRUCTIONS:

1. Preheat oven to 375°F.
2. Place salmon fillets on a lined baking sheet.
3. In a small bowl, mix olive oil, lemon zest, juice, thyme, salt, and pepper.
4. Brush mixture over salmon.
5. Bake for 12–15 minutes or until cooked through.

Nutrition:

Calories: 320 | **Protein:** 28g | **Fat:** 20g | **Carbohydrates:** 1g | **Fiber:** 0g

Turmeric Chicken Stir-Fry

Prep Time: 10 minutes + 10 minutes cooking

Serves: 2

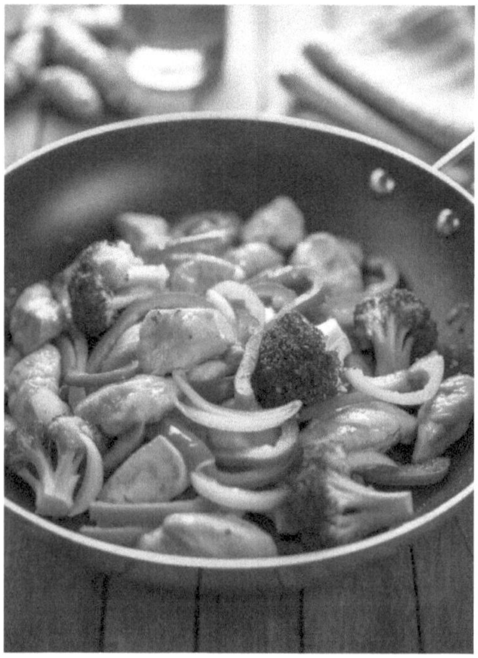

INGREDIENTS:

- 1 chicken breast, sliced
- 1 tbsp olive oil
- 1/2 cup bell pepper strips
- 1/2 cup broccoli florets
- 1/4 cup sliced onion
- 1/2 tsp ground turmeric
- Salt and pepper to taste

INSTRUCTIONS:

1. Heat olive oil in a skillet over medium heat.
2. Add chicken and cook until browned, about 4–5 minutes.
3. Add vegetables and turmeric. Stir-fry for 5 more minutes.
4. Season to taste and serve hot.

Nutrition:

Calories: 290 | **Protein:** 27g | **Fat:** 16g | **Carbohydrates:** 8g | **Fiber:** 2g | **Anti-Inflammatory:** High | **Vitamin C:** Moderate

Grilled Sardine Lettuce Wraps

Prep Time: 10 minutes

Serves: 2

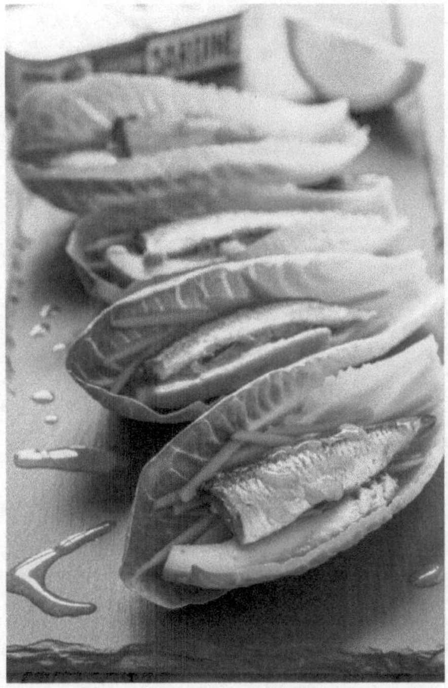

INGREDIENTS:

- 1 can sardines in olive oil, drained
- 4 large romaine or butter lettuce leaves
- 1/2 avocado, sliced
- 1/4 cup shredded carrots
- 1 tsp lemon juice
- Salt and pepper to taste

INSTRUCTIONS:

1. Place sardines, avocado, and carrots in the center of each lettuce leaf.
2. Drizzle with lemon juice and season.
3. Roll or fold lettuce around the filling and serve.

Nutrition:

Calories: 270 | **Protein:** 18g | **Fat:** 20g | **Carbohydrates:** 6g | **Fiber:** 4g

Rosemary Garlic Chicken Thighs

Prep Time: 10 minutes + 20 minutes baking

Serves: 2

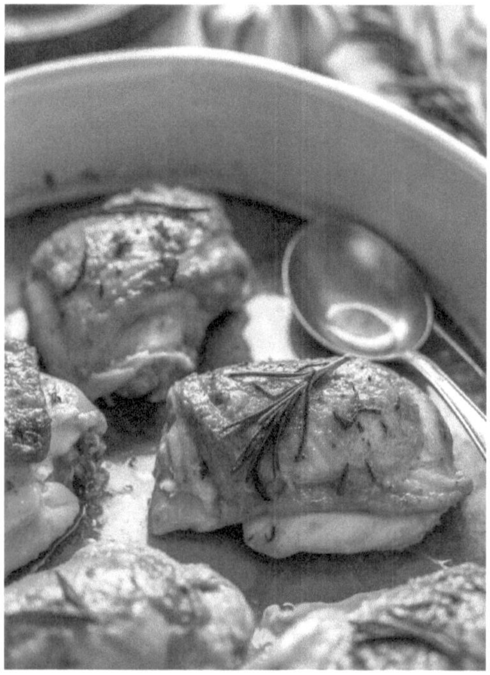

INGREDIENTS:

- 2 boneless, skinless chicken thighs
- 1 tbsp olive oil
- 1 garlic clove, minced
- 1/2 tsp dried rosemary
- Salt and pepper to taste

INSTRUCTIONS:

1. Preheat oven to 400°F.
2. In a bowl, mix olive oil, garlic, rosemary, salt, and pepper.
3. Rub mixture over chicken and place in a baking dish.
4. Bake for 18–20 minutes or until fully cooked.

Nutrition:

Calories: 280 | **Protein:** 26g | **Fat:** 18g | **Carbohydrates:** 1g | **Fiber:** 0g | **B Vitamins:** High | **Anti-Inflammatory:** Moderate

Tuna & White Bean Salad

Prep Time: 10 minutes

Serves: 2

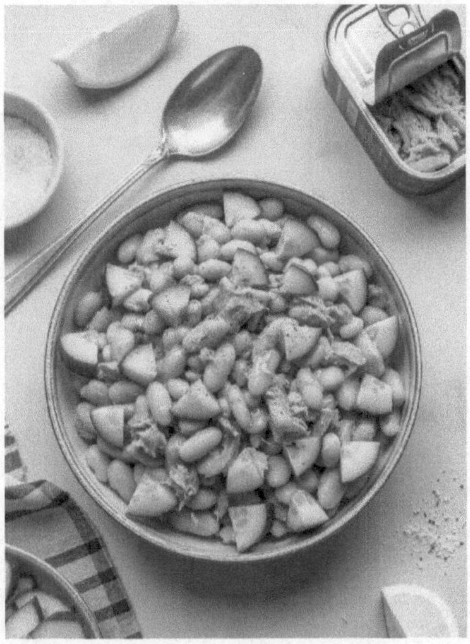

INGREDIENTS:

- 1 can tuna in water, drained
- 1/2 cup canned white beans, rinsed
- 1/4 cup diced cucumber
- 1 tbsp olive oil
- 1 tsp lemon juice
- Salt and pepper to taste

INSTRUCTIONS:

1. In a bowl, mix tuna, white beans, and cucumber.
2. Drizzle with olive oil and lemon juice.
3. Toss gently and season to taste.
4. Serve chilled or at room temperature.

Nutrition:

Calories: 250 | **Protein:** 22g | **Fat:** 10g | **Carbohydrates:** 14g | **Fiber:** 3g

25. PLANT-BASED MAINS FOR MOOD SUPPORT

Sweet Potato & Black Bean Tacos

Prep Time: 15 minutes

Serves: 2

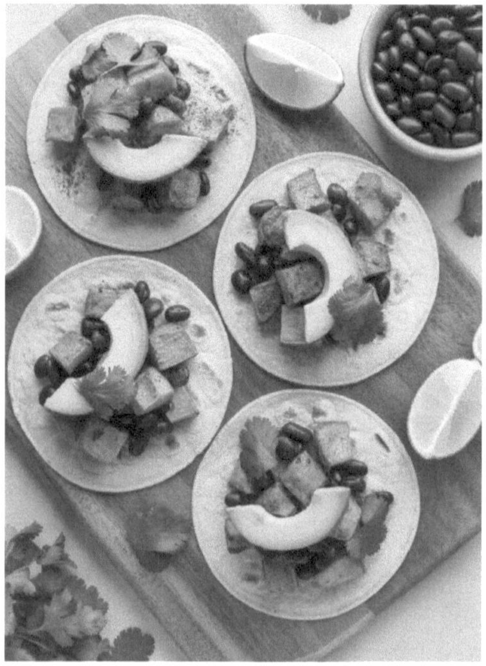

INGREDIENTS:

- 1 medium sweet potato, peeled and diced
- 1/2 cup canned black beans, rinsed
- 1/4 tsp cumin
- 1/4 tsp paprika
- 1 tbsp olive oil
- 4 small corn tortillas
- 1/4 avocado, sliced

INSTRUCTIONS:

1. Preheat oven to 400°F.
2. Toss sweet potato with olive oil, cumin, and paprika. Roast for 20 minutes.
3. Warm tortillas and fill with sweet potato, black beans, and avocado.
4. Serve warm.

Nutrition:

Calories: 320 | **Protein:** 10g | **Fat:** 12g | **Carbohydrates:** 44g | **Fiber:** 9g

Chickpea & Spinach Coconut Curry

Prep Time: 10 minutes + 15 minutes simmer

Serves: 2

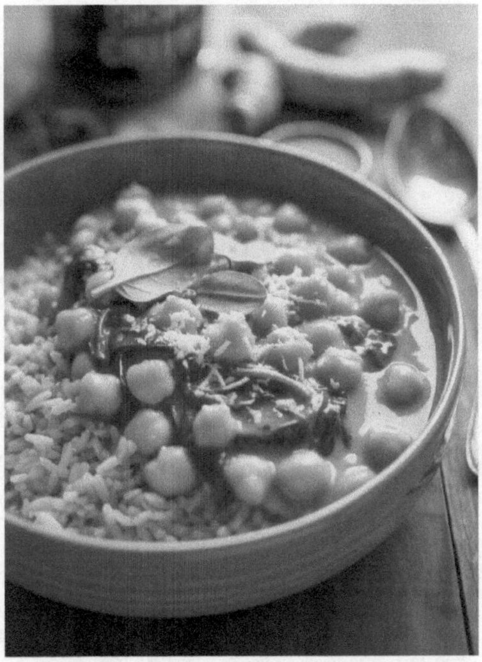

INGREDIENTS:

- 1 tbsp olive oil
- 1/2 onion, diced
- 1 garlic clove, minced
- 1/2 tsp curry powder
- 1/2 can coconut milk
- 1/2 can chickpeas, rinsed
- 1 cup fresh spinach
- Salt to taste

INSTRUCTIONS:

1. Heat oil in a skillet and sauté onion and garlic for 3–4 minutes.
2. Stir in curry powder, chickpeas, and coconut milk. Simmer for 10 minutes.
3. Add spinach and cook until wilted.
4. Season and serve warm over brown rice if desired.

Nutrition:

Calories: 290 | **Protein:** 9g | **Fat:** 18g | **Carbohydrates:** 22g | **Fiber:** 5g

Lentil Mushroom Shepherd's Pie

Prep Time: 20 minutes + 20 minutes baking

Serves: 4

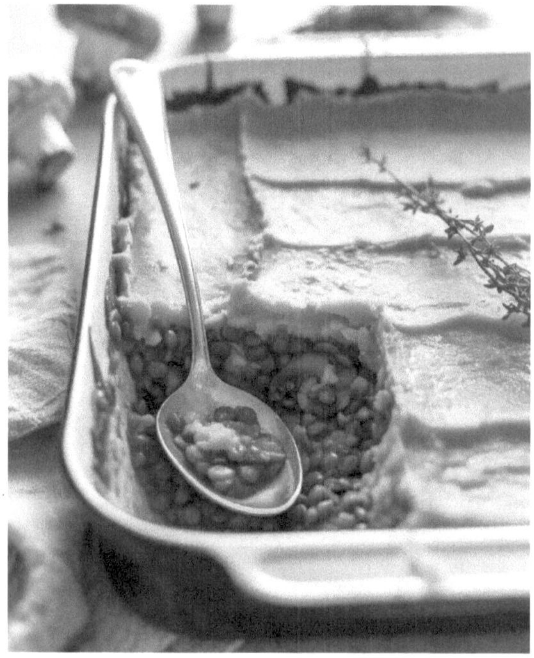

INGREDIENTS:

- 1 cup cooked green lentils
- 1 cup mushrooms, chopped
- 1/2 onion, diced
- 1/2 cup peas
- 2 cups mashed sweet potatoes
- 1 tbsp olive oil
- Salt and herbs to taste

INSTRUCTIONS:

1. Preheat oven to 375°F.
2. Heat oil in a skillet and sauté onion and mushrooms until soft.
3. Stir in lentils, peas, salt, and herbs.
4. Spread mixture into a baking dish and top with mashed sweet potatoes.
5. Bake for 20 minutes or until warmed through.

Nutrition:

Calories: 330 | **Protein:** 13g | **Fat:** 9g | **Carbohydrates:** 47g | **Fiber:** 10g | **Serotonin Support:** High | **Vitamin B6:** Moderate

Tofu Stir-Fry with Broccoli & Cashews

Prep Time: 15 minutes

Serves: 2

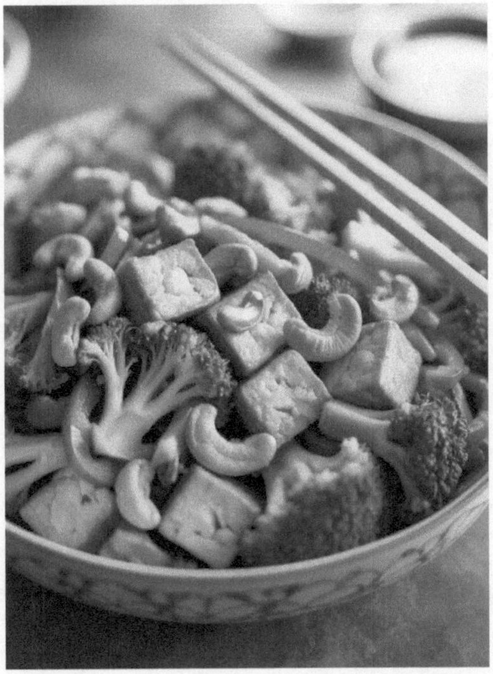

INGREDIENTS:

- 1/2 block firm tofu, cubed
- 1 tbsp olive or sesame oil
- 1 cup broccoli florets
- 1/2 bell pepper, sliced
- 1/4 cup cashews
- 1 tbsp low-sodium soy sauce

INSTRUCTIONS:

1. Heat oil in a skillet and cook tofu until golden. Remove and set aside.
2. In the same pan, stir-fry broccoli and bell pepper for 5–6 minutes.
3. Add tofu back in along with soy sauce and cashews. Stir well.
4. Serve over brown rice or quinoa.

Nutrition:

Calories: 340 | **Protein:** 14g | **Fat:** 20g | **Carbohydrates:** 22g | **Fiber:** 5g

Stuffed Bell Peppers with Quinoa & Walnuts

Prep Time: 20 minutes + 25 minutes baking

Serves: 2

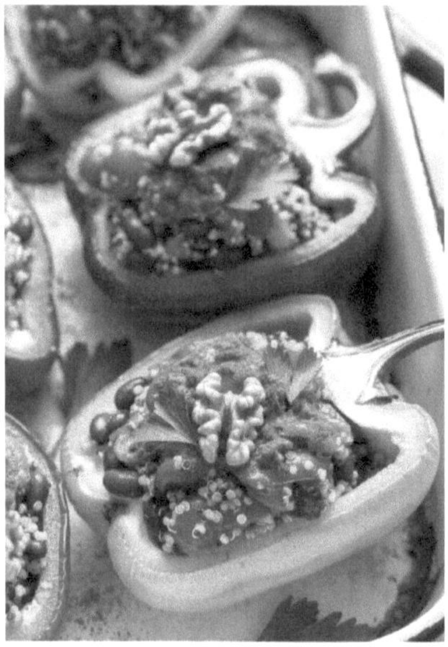

INGREDIENTS:

- 2 bell peppers, halved and seeded
- 1/2 cup cooked quinoa
- 1/4 cup chopped walnuts
- 1/4 cup black beans
- 1/4 cup diced tomato
- 1 tbsp olive oil
- Salt, cumin, and paprika to taste

INSTRUCTIONS:

1. Preheat oven to 375°F.
2. Mix quinoa, walnuts, beans, tomato, olive oil, and spices.
3. Spoon the mixture into bell pepper halves.
4. Bake in a dish covered with foil for 20 minutes. Remove foil and bake 5 more minutes.
5. Serve warm.

Nutrition:

Calories: 310 | **Protein:** 10g | **Fat:** 16g | **Carbohydrates:** 34g | **Fiber:** 8g | **Plant-Based Omega-3s:** Moderate | **Brain-Soothing Ingredients:** Yes

Let me know when you're ready for **Section 26: Low-Sodium Comfort Food Classics** or another part of the book!

26. LOW-SODIUM COMFORT FOOD CLASSICS

Vegetable Lentil Loaf

Prep Time: 15 minutes + 40 minutes baking

Serves: 4

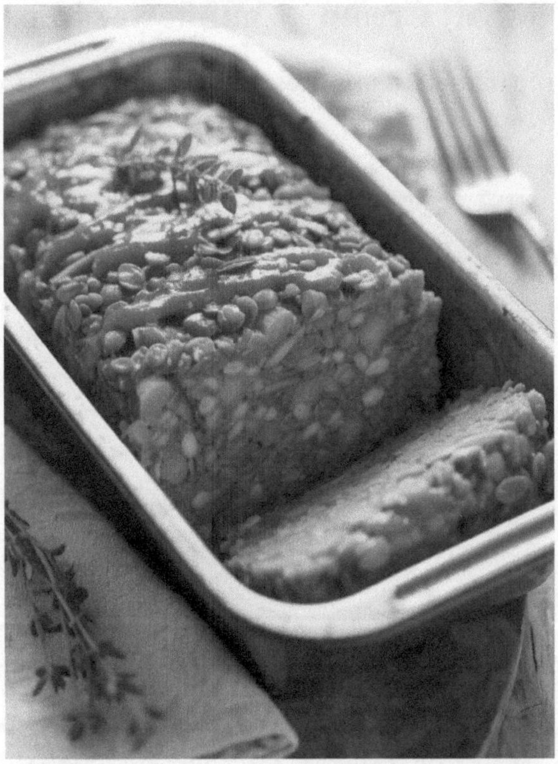

INGREDIENTS:

- 1 cup cooked lentils
- 1/2 cup oats
- 1/4 cup grated carrot
- 1/4 cup finely chopped onion
- 1 tbsp ground flaxseed
- 2 tbsp tomato paste (no salt added)
- 1 tsp garlic powder
- 1/2 tsp thyme

INSTRUCTIONS:

1. Preheat oven to 375°F.
2. In a bowl, mix all ingredients until well combined.
3. Press mixture into a greased loaf pan.
4. Bake for 35–40 minutes or until firm.

5. Let cool slightly before slicing and serving.

Nutrition:

Calories: 230 | **Protein:** 11g | **Fat:** 6g | **Carbohydrates:** 32g | **Fiber:** 8g

No-Salt Creamy Cauliflower Mash

Prep Time: 10 minutes + 10 minutes cooking

Serves: 2

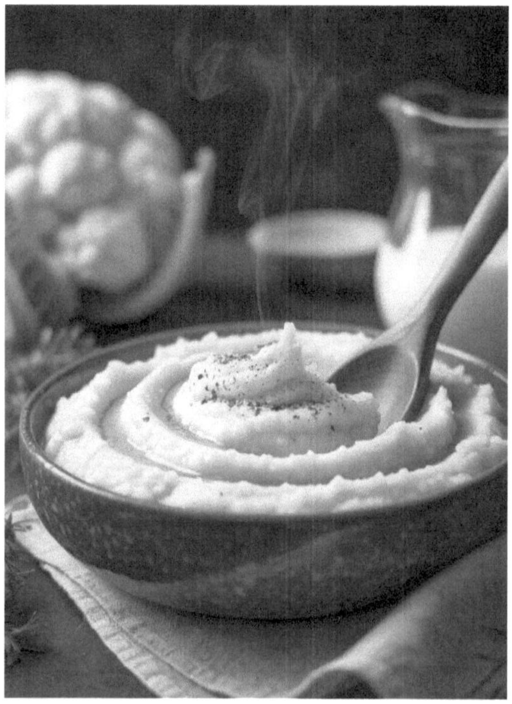

INGREDIENTS:

- 2 cups cauliflower florets
- 1 tbsp olive oil
- 1/4 cup unsweetened almond milk
- 1/4 tsp garlic powder
- Black pepper to taste

INSTRUCTIONS:

1. Steam cauliflower until very tender.
2. Transfer to a food processor with olive oil, almond milk, and garlic powder.
3. Blend until smooth.
4. Season with black pepper and serve warm.

Nutrition:

Calories: 120 | **Protein:** 3g | **Fat:** 9g | **Carbohydrates:** 9g | **Fiber:** 3g

Stuffed Zucchini Boats

Prep Time: 15 minutes + 20 minutes baking

Serves: 2

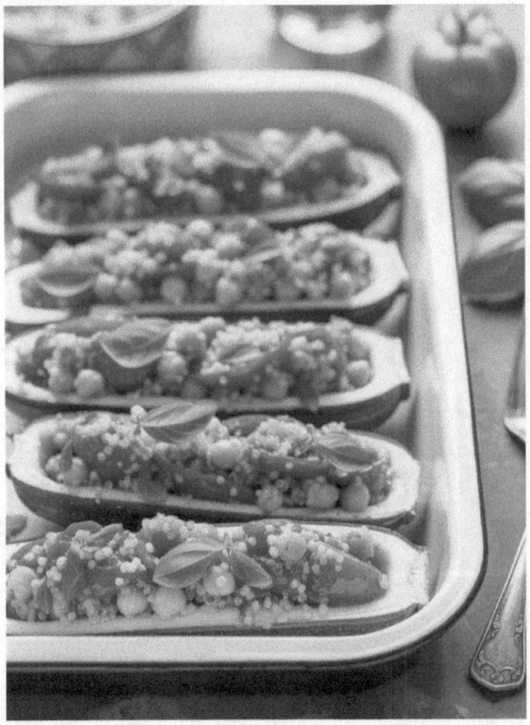

INGREDIENTS:

- 2 medium zucchinis, halved lengthwise and scooped
- 1/2 cup cooked quinoa
- 1/4 cup diced tomatoes
- 1/4 cup chickpeas
- 1 tbsp olive oil
- 1/2 tsp dried basil
- Pepper to taste

INSTRUCTIONS:

1. Preheat oven to 375°F.
2. Mix quinoa, tomatoes, chickpeas, oil, basil, and pepper in a bowl.
3. Fill zucchini halves with mixture.
4. Bake in a dish for 20 minutes or until zucchini is tender.

Nutrition:

Calories: 210 | **Protein:** 7g | **Fat:** 10g | **Carbohydrates:** 22g | **Fiber:** 5g

Low-Sodium Mushroom Stroganoff

Prep Time: 15 minutes

Serves: 2

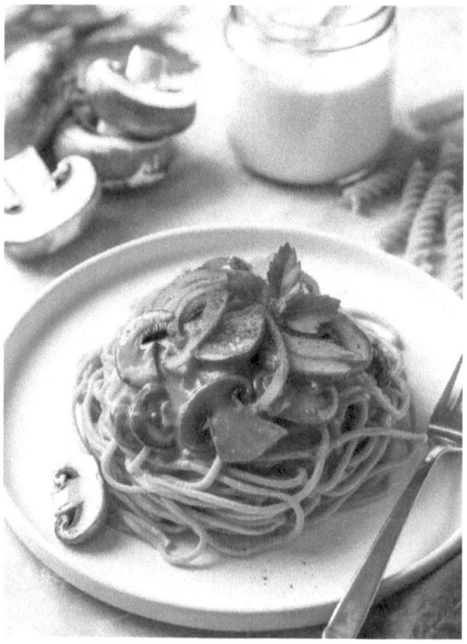

INGREDIENTS:

- 2 cups sliced mushrooms
- 1/2 onion, chopped
- 1 tbsp olive oil
- 1/2 cup plain Greek yogurt
- 1/2 tsp paprika
- 1/2 tsp garlic powder
- 1 cup whole wheat pasta, cooked
- Black pepper to taste

INSTRUCTIONS:

1. Heat oil in a skillet and sauté onions and mushrooms until soft.
2. Stir in garlic powder and paprika.
3. Remove from heat and mix in yogurt.
4. Serve over warm pasta and season with pepper.

Nutrition:

Calories: 310 | **Protein:** 12g | **Fat:** 12g | **Carbohydrates:** 36g | **Fiber:** 6g

Sweet Potato & Kale Skillet Hash

Prep Time: 10 minutes + 15 minutes cooking

Serves: 2

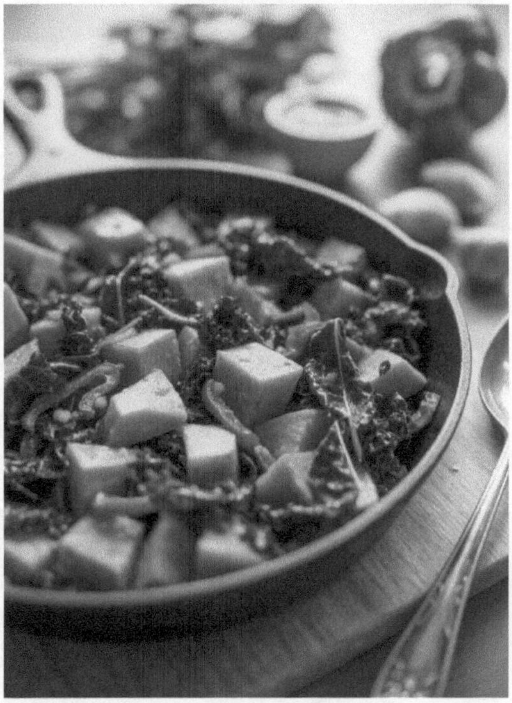

INGREDIENTS:

- 1 medium sweet potato, diced
- 1 cup chopped kale
- 1/4 cup diced red bell pepper
- 1 tbsp olive oil
- 1/2 tsp cumin
- Black pepper to taste

INSTRUCTIONS:

1. Heat olive oil in a skillet over medium heat.
2. Add sweet potato and cook for 8–10 minutes until soft.
3. Stir in kale, bell pepper, cumin, and pepper.
4. Cook 5 more minutes and serve warm.

Nutrition:

Calories: 250 | **Protein:** 5g | **Fat:** 11g | **Carbohydrates:** 33g | **Fiber:** 7g

27. ONE-PAN MEALS FOR EASY CLEANUP

Mediterranean Chickpea Sheet Pan Bake

Prep Time: 10 minutes + 25 minutes baking

Serves: 3

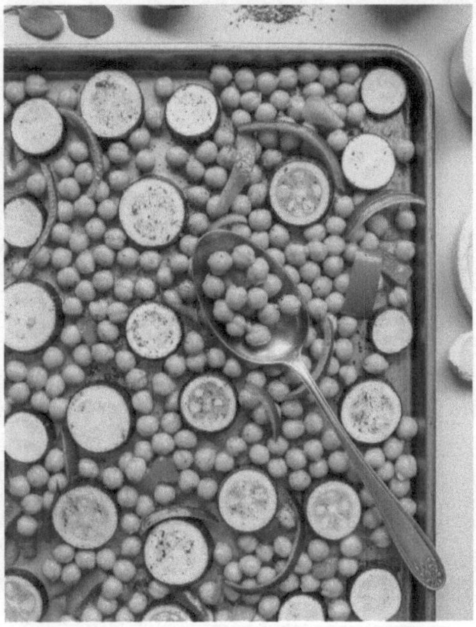

INGREDIENTS:

- 1 can chickpeas, rinsed and drained
- 1 zucchini, sliced
- 1 bell pepper, chopped
- 1/2 red onion, sliced
- 2 tbsp olive oil
- 1 tsp oregano
- 1/2 tsp garlic powder
- Pepper to taste

INSTRUCTIONS:

1. Preheat oven to 400°F.
2. On a sheet pan, toss all ingredients together to coat evenly.
3. Spread in a single layer and bake for 25 minutes, stirring halfway through.
4. Serve warm or store for easy reheating.

Nutrition:

Calories: 310 | **Protein:** 11g | **Fat:** 14g | **Carbohydrates:** 36g | **Fiber:** 10g

Salmon & Veggie Foil Packets

Prep Time: 10 minutes + 20 minutes baking

Serves: 2

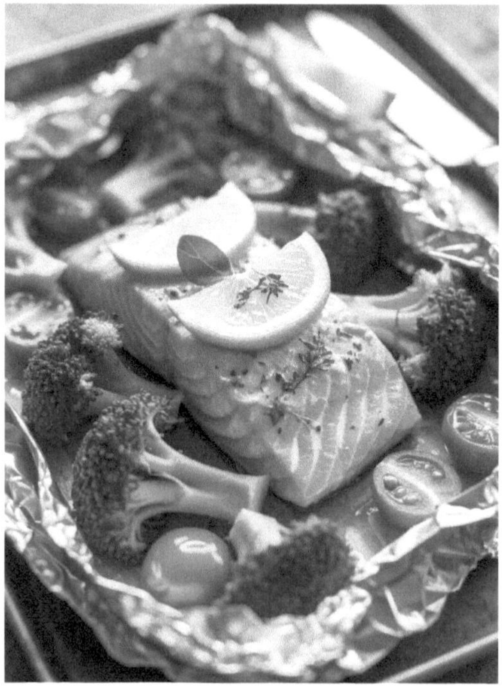

INGREDIENTS:

- 2 salmon fillets
- 1 cup broccoli florets
- 1/2 cup cherry tomatoes
- 1 tbsp olive oil
- 1/2 lemon, sliced
- 1/2 tsp dill or parsley
- Pepper to taste

INSTRUCTIONS:

1. Preheat oven to 375°F.
2. Place salmon and vegetables in foil sheets.
3. Drizzle with olive oil and season with herbs and pepper.
4. Top with lemon slices, seal packets, and bake for 20 minutes.
5. Serve directly in the foil for easy cleanup.

Nutrition:

Calories: 350 | **Protein:** 30g | **Fat:** 22g | **Carbohydrates:** 8g | **Fiber:** 3g

One-Pan Tofu Stir-Fry Bowl

Prep Time: 10 minutes + 10 minutes cooking

Serves: 2

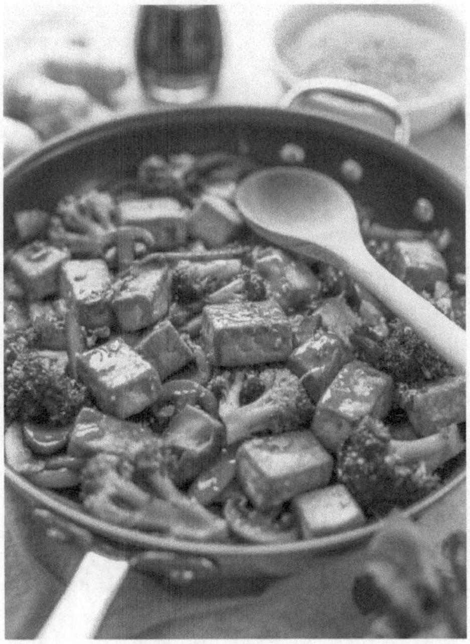

INGREDIENTS:

- 1/2 block firm tofu, cubed
- 1 cup chopped broccoli
- 1/2 cup sliced mushrooms
- 1/2 bell pepper, chopped
- 1 tbsp olive or sesame oil
- 1 tbsp low-sodium soy sauce
- 1/2 tsp ginger powder

INSTRUCTIONS:

1. Heat oil in a skillet over medium heat.
2. Add tofu and cook until golden, about 5 minutes.
3. Add vegetables, soy sauce, and ginger. Stir and cook for 5 more minutes.
4. Serve hot over whole grain rice or quinoa.

Nutrition:

Calories: 300 | **Protein:** 14g | **Fat:** 17g | **Carbohydrates:** 24g | **Fiber:** 5g

Balsamic Chicken & Veggie Skillet

Prep Time: 10 minutes + 15 minutes cooking

Serves: 2

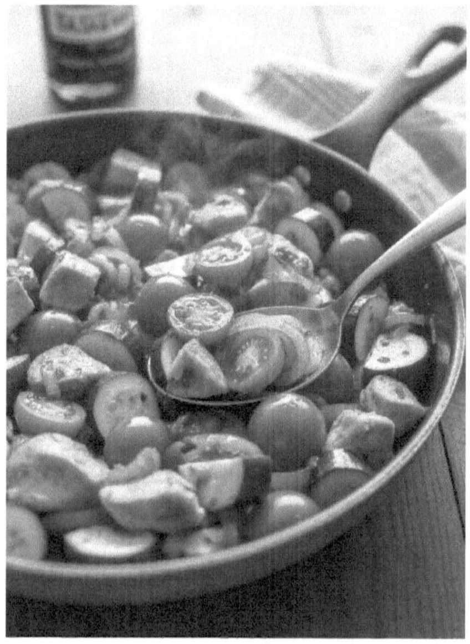

INGREDIENTS:

- 1 chicken breast, cubed
- 1/2 zucchini, chopped
- 1/2 cup grape tomatoes
- 1/4 onion, sliced
- 1 tbsp olive oil
- 1 tbsp balsamic vinegar
- 1/2 tsp basil

INSTRUCTIONS:

1. Heat olive oil in a skillet.
2. Add chicken and cook until browned, about 6 minutes.
3. Add vegetables, vinegar, and basil. Stir and cook 8–10 more minutes.
4. Serve directly from skillet.

Nutrition:

Calories: 330 | **Protein:** 26g | **Fat:** 16g | **Carbohydrates:** 14g | **Fiber:** 3g

Eggplant & Chickpea Tomato Bake

Prep Time: 10 minutes + 25 minutes baking

Serves: 3

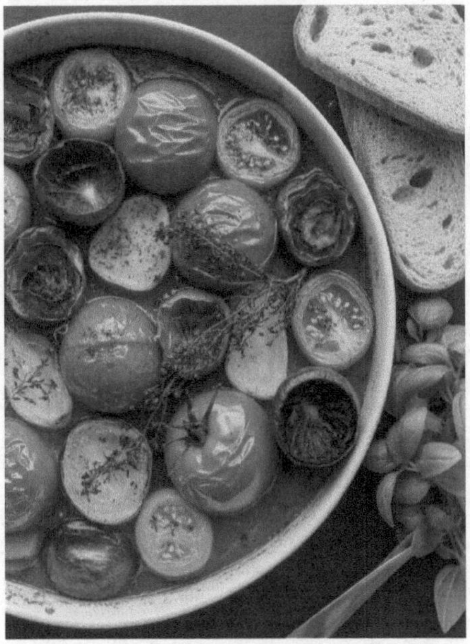

INGREDIENTS:

- 1 small eggplant, cubed
- 1 can chickpeas, rinsed
- 1/2 cup diced tomatoes (no salt added)
- 1/4 cup chopped red onion
- 1 tbsp olive oil
- 1 tsp cumin
- 1/2 tsp smoked paprika

INSTRUCTIONS:

1. Preheat oven to 400°F.
2. In a baking dish, toss all ingredients together.
3. Spread evenly and bake for 25 minutes, stirring halfway through.
4. Serve warm from the dish.

Nutrition:

Calories: 280 | **Protein:** 10g | **Fat:** 10g | **Carbohydrates:** 36g | **Fiber:** 9g

28. ANTI-INFLAMMATORY PASTA & GRAIN DISHES

Turmeric Quinoa & Roasted Veggie Bowl

Prep Time: 10 minutes + 25 minutes roasting

Serves: 2

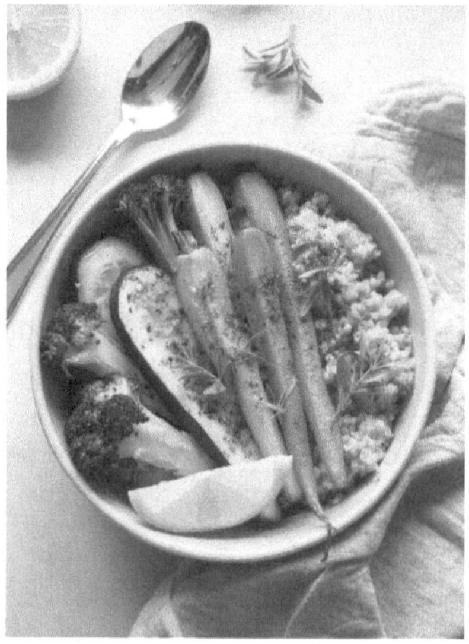

INGREDIENTS:

- 1/2 cup cooked quinoa
- 1 cup chopped vegetables (carrot, broccoli, zucchini)
- 1 tbsp olive oil
- 1/2 tsp turmeric
- 1/4 tsp black pepper
- 1/2 tsp cumin

INSTRUCTIONS:

1. Preheat oven to 400°F.
2. Toss vegetables with olive oil, turmeric, pepper, and cumin.
3. Spread on a baking sheet and roast for 25 minutes.
4. Serve over cooked quinoa and enjoy warm.

Nutrition:

Calories: 280 | **Protein:** 9g | **Fat:** 14g | **Carbohydrates:** 30g | **Fiber:** 6g | **Anti-Inflammatory:** High | **Brain Nourishing:** Yes

Whole Wheat Pasta with Garlic Kale & Walnuts

Prep Time: 15 minutes

Serves: 2

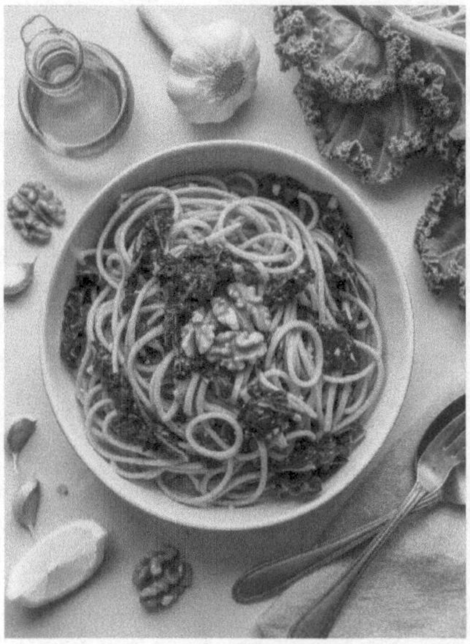

INGREDIENTS:

- 1 cup cooked whole wheat pasta
- 2 cups kale, chopped
- 2 garlic cloves, minced
- 1 tbsp olive oil
- 2 tbsp chopped walnuts
- 1/2 tsp lemon juice

INSTRUCTIONS:

1. In a skillet, heat olive oil and sauté garlic for 1 minute.
2. Add kale and cook until wilted, about 5 minutes.
3. Add pasta, walnuts, and lemon juice. Stir well and serve warm.

Nutrition:

Calories: 330 | **Protein:** 11g | **Fat:** 15g | **Carbohydrates:** 38g | **Fiber:** 7g

Barley & Tomato Warm Salad

Prep Time: 20 minutes

Serves: 2

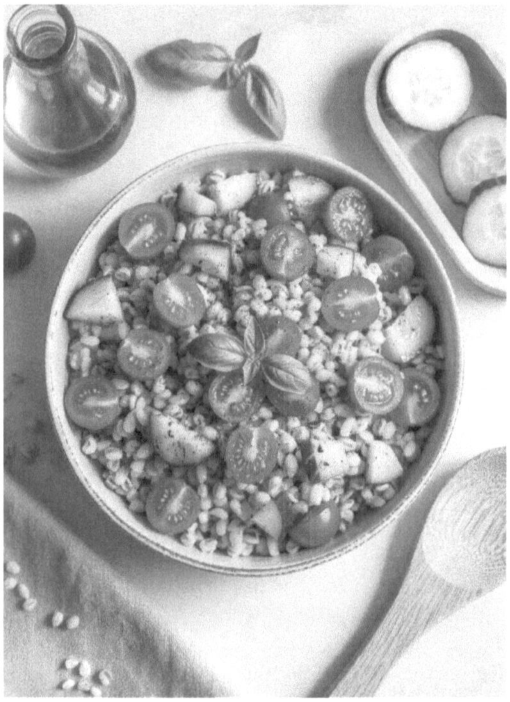

INGREDIENTS:

- 1/2 cup cooked pearl barley
- 1/2 cup cherry tomatoes, halved
- 1/4 cup cucumber, chopped
- 1 tbsp olive oil
- 1/2 tsp dried basil
- 1 tsp apple cider vinegar

INSTRUCTIONS:

1. In a bowl, combine barley, tomatoes, and cucumber.
2. Drizzle with olive oil and vinegar.
3. Add basil, toss well, and serve slightly warm or room temperature.

Nutrition:

Calories: 250 | **Protein:** 6g | **Fat:** 10g | **Carbohydrates:** 35g | **Fiber:** 5g

Spiced Lentil Pasta with Spinach

Prep Time: 15 minutes

Serves: 2

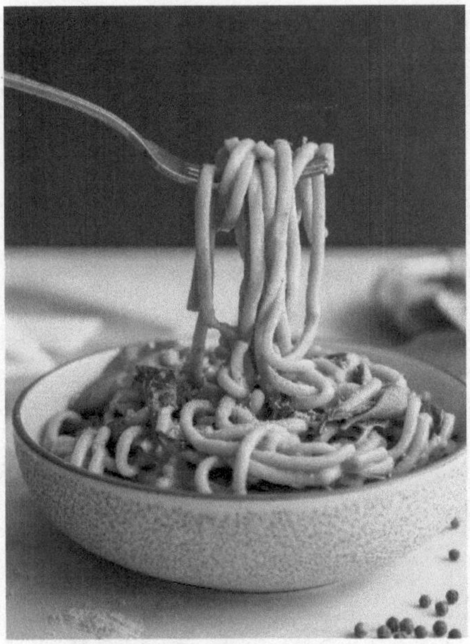

INGREDIENTS:

- 1 cup cooked lentil or chickpea pasta
- 1 cup fresh spinach
- 1 tbsp olive oil
- 1/2 tsp turmeric
- 1/4 tsp black pepper
- 1 tbsp nutritional yeast or grated cheese

INSTRUCTIONS:

1. In a skillet, heat olive oil and add turmeric and pepper.
2. Stir in spinach and cook until wilted.
3. Toss in cooked pasta and nutritional yeast. Mix and serve.

Nutrition:

Calories: 310 | **Protein:** 16g | **Fat:** 11g | **Carbohydrates:** 32g | **Fiber:** 8g

Farro & Roasted Beet Bowl

Prep Time: 10 minutes + 25 minutes roasting

Serves: 2

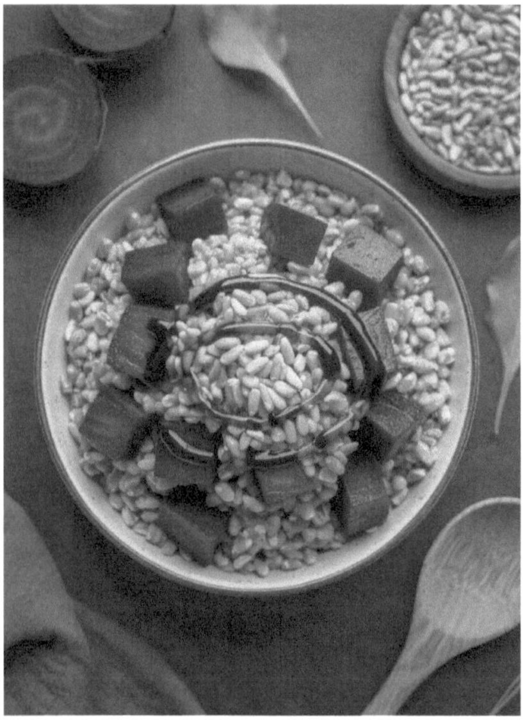

INGREDIENTS:

- 1/2 cup cooked farro
- 1 medium beet, peeled and diced
- 1 tbsp olive oil
- 1 tbsp sunflower seeds
- 1 tsp balsamic vinegar

INSTRUCTIONS:

1. Preheat oven to 400°F.
2. Toss beets with olive oil and roast for 25 minutes.
3. Combine cooked farro and roasted beets in a bowl.
4. Add sunflower seeds and drizzle with balsamic vinegar. Serve warm.

Nutrition:

Calories: 290 | **Protein:** 8g | **Fat:** 13g | **Carbohydrates:** 35g | **Fiber:** 6g

29. LIGHT & NOURISHING DINNERS

Lemon Herb Baked Salmon

Prep Time: 20 minutes

Serves: 2

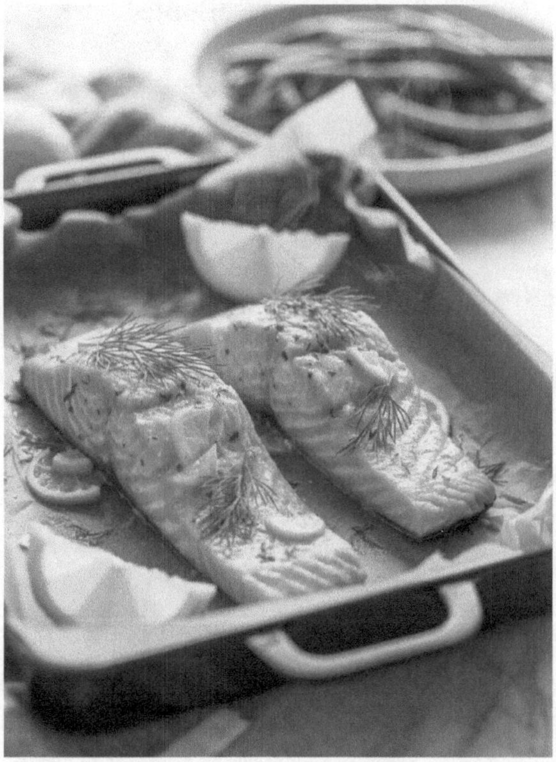

INGREDIENTS:

- 2 salmon fillets (4 oz each)
- 1 tbsp olive oil
- Juice of 1/2 lemon
- 1 garlic clove, minced
- 1 tsp chopped fresh dill or parsley
- Salt and pepper to taste

INSTRUCTIONS:

1. Preheat oven to 375°F.
2. Place salmon fillets on a parchment-lined baking dish.
3. In a small bowl, whisk olive oil, lemon juice, garlic, herbs, salt, and pepper.
4. Pour mixture over salmon and bake for 15–18 minutes or until fish flakes easily.
5. Serve with steamed vegetables or a side salad.

Nutrition:

Calories: 280 | **Protein:** 26g | **Fat:** 18g | **Carbohydrates:** 2g

Zucchini Noodle Stir-Fry

Prep Time: 15 minutes

Serves: 2

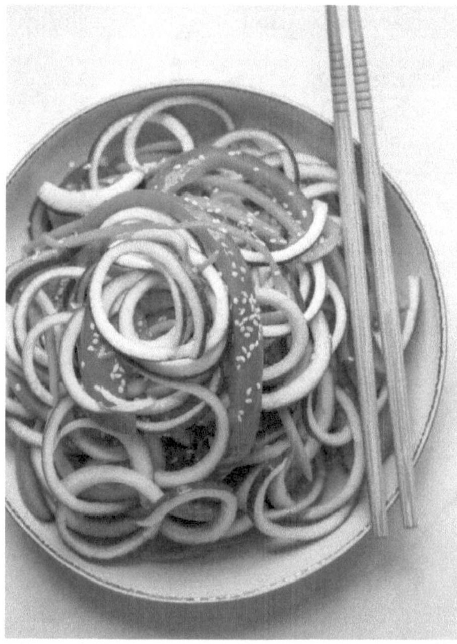

INGREDIENTS:

- 2 medium zucchinis, spiralized
- 1/2 red bell pepper, sliced
- 1/2 cup shredded carrots
- 1 tbsp low-sodium soy sauce
- 1 tsp sesame oil
- 1 tsp olive oil
- 1 tsp minced ginger

INSTRUCTIONS:

1. Heat olive oil in a skillet over medium heat.
2. Add ginger, bell pepper, and carrots. Cook for 3 minutes.
3. Add zucchini noodles and sauté for another 2–3 minutes.
4. Stir in soy sauce and sesame oil. Cook for 1 more minute.

5. Serve warm as a light dinner or side dish.

Nutrition:

Calories: 150 | **Protein:** 3g | **Fat:** 8g | **Carbohydrates:** 14g | **Fiber:** 4g

Mediterranean Chickpea Salad

Prep Time: 10 minutes

Serves: 2

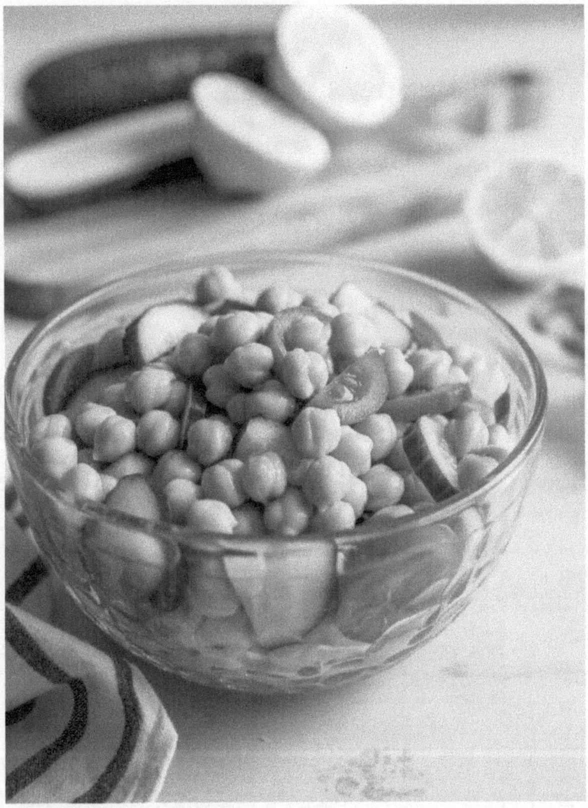

INGREDIENTS:

- 1 cup canned chickpeas, rinsed and drained
- 1/2 cup cherry tomatoes, halved
- 1/2 cucumber, diced
- 1/4 cup red onion, finely chopped
- 1 tbsp olive oil
- 1 tbsp lemon juice
- 1 tbsp chopped parsley
- Salt and pepper to taste

INSTRUCTIONS:

1. Combine chickpeas, tomatoes, cucumber, and onion in a bowl.
2. Drizzle with olive oil and lemon juice.
3. Add parsley, salt, and pepper. Toss gently.
4. Chill for 10 minutes before serving for best flavor.

Nutrition:

Calories: 220 | **Protein:** 8g | **Fat:** 10g | **Carbohydrates:** 24g | **Fiber:** 6g

Stuffed Bell Peppers with Quinoa & Spinach

Prep Time: 25 minutes

Serves: 2

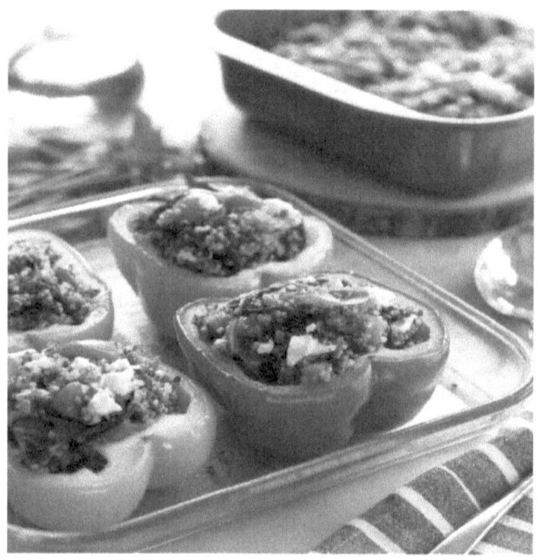

INGREDIENTS:

- 2 bell peppers, halved and seeded
- 1/2 cup cooked quinoa
- 1 cup spinach, chopped
- 1/4 cup diced tomatoes
- 2 tbsp crumbled feta cheese
- 1 tbsp olive oil
- Salt and pepper to taste

INSTRUCTIONS:

1. Preheat oven to 375°F.
2. In a skillet, sauté spinach in olive oil until wilted.

3. Mix spinach with quinoa, tomatoes, feta, salt, and pepper.
4. Fill bell pepper halves with mixture and place in a baking dish.
5. Bake for 15–20 minutes until peppers are tender.

Nutrition:

Calories: 260 | **Protein:** 9g | **Fat:** 13g | **Carbohydrates:** 25g | **Fiber:** 5g

Herbed Lentil & Veggie Stew

Prep Time: 30 minutes

Serves: 3

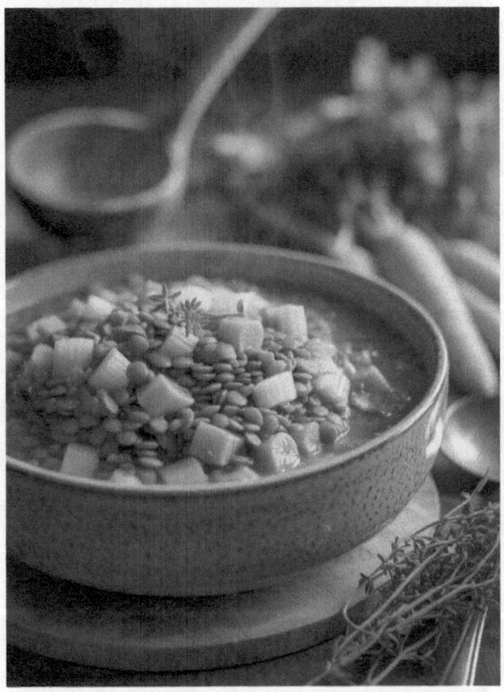

INGREDIENTS:

- 1/2 cup dried lentils, rinsed
- 1 carrot, diced
- 1 celery stalk, diced
- 1/2 onion, chopped
- 2 cups low-sodium vegetable broth
- 1 tsp olive oil
- 1/2 tsp thyme
- Salt and pepper to taste

INSTRUCTIONS:

1. Heat olive oil in a pot and sauté onion, carrot, and celery for 5 minutes.
2. Add lentils, broth, thyme, salt, and pepper. Bring to a boil.
3. Reduce heat and simmer uncovered for 20–25 minutes until lentils are tender.
4. Stir and serve warm.

Nutrition:

Calories: 230 | **Protein:** 12g | **Fat:** 5g | **Carbohydrates:** 35g | **Fiber:** 9g

30. MEMORY-BOOSTING CASSEROLES

Spinach & Mushroom Egg Bake

Prep Time: 15 minutes

Serves: 4

INGREDIENTS:

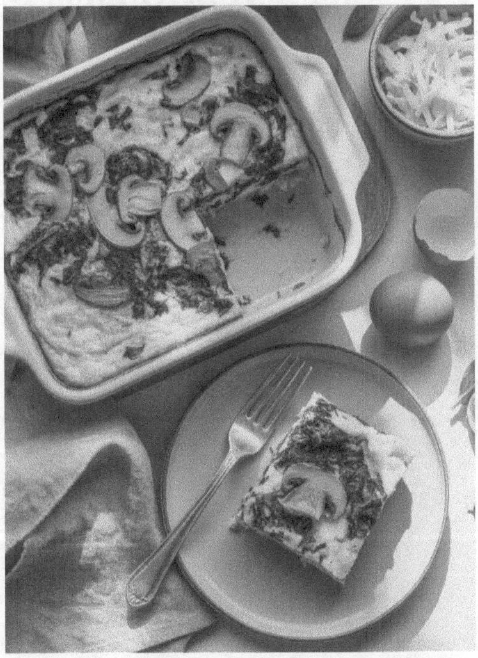

- 6 eggs
- 1 cup chopped spinach
- 1/2 cup sliced mushrooms
- 1/4 cup diced onion
- 1/4 cup shredded mozzarella
- 1/4 cup milk or milk alternative
- 1 tbsp olive oil
- Salt and pepper to taste

INSTRUCTIONS:

1. Preheat oven to 375°F.
2. Sauté mushrooms and onion in olive oil for 3–4 minutes.
3. In a large bowl, whisk eggs, milk, salt, and pepper.
4. Stir in spinach, cooked veggies, and cheese.
5. Pour mixture into a greased 8x8 baking dish.

6. Bake for 20–25 minutes until center is set.
7. Cool slightly before slicing and serving.

Nutrition:

Calories: 210 | **Protein:** 14g | **Fat:** 15g | **Carbohydrates:** 4g | **Fiber:** 1g

Sweet Potato & Kale Quinoa Bake

Prep Time: 20 minutes

Serves: 4

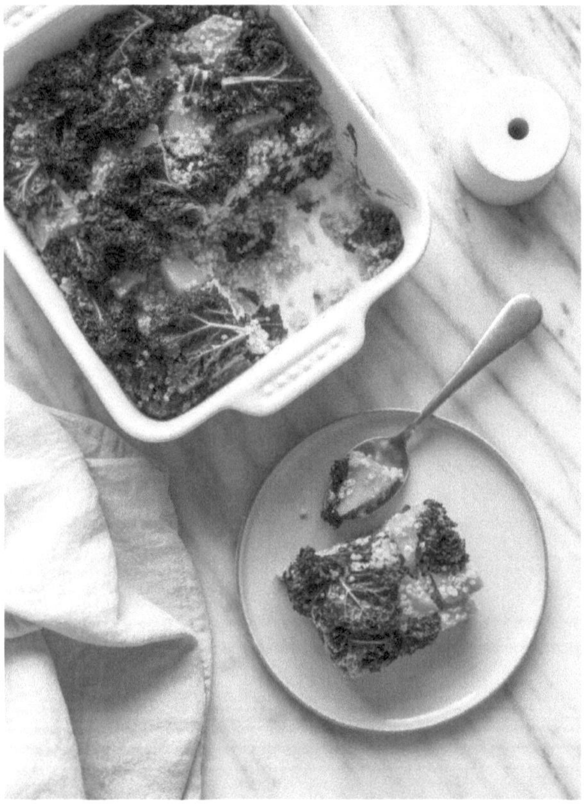

INGREDIENTS:

- 1 cup cooked quinoa
- 1 cup chopped kale
- 1 cup diced cooked sweet potato
- 1/4 cup crumbled feta cheese
- 2 eggs
- 1/4 cup milk
- 1 tsp olive oil
- Salt and pepper to taste

INSTRUCTIONS:

1. Preheat oven to 375°F.
2. In a skillet, sauté kale in olive oil for 2–3 minutes.
3. In a bowl, combine quinoa, sweet potato, kale, feta, eggs, milk, salt, and pepper.
4. Mix well and spread into a greased 9-inch baking dish.
5. Bake for 25–30 minutes until golden on top and set.

Nutrition:

Calories: 250 | **Protein:** 11g | **Fat:** 12g | **Carbohydrates:** 24g | **Fiber:** 4g

Broccoli Chickpea Casserole

Prep Time: 15 minutes

Serves: 4

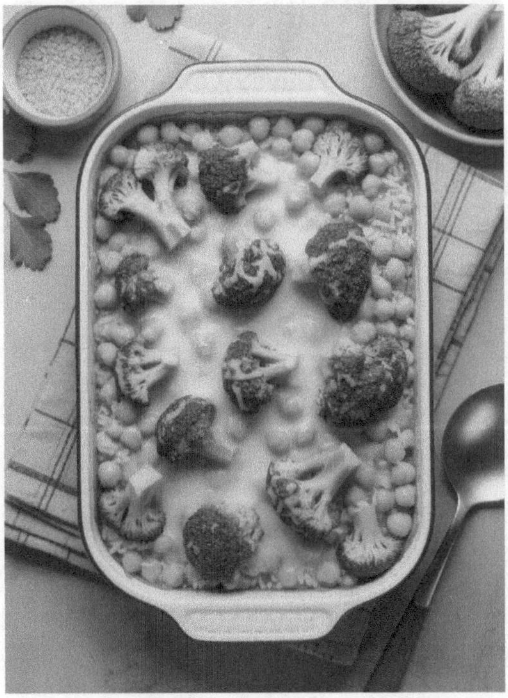

INGREDIENTS:

- 1 can chickpeas, drained and rinsed
- 1 cup chopped steamed broccoli
- 1/2 cup cooked brown rice
- 1/4 cup plain Greek yogurt
- 1/4 cup shredded cheddar or plant-based cheese

- 1 tbsp olive oil
- 1/2 tsp garlic powder
- Salt and pepper to taste

INSTRUCTIONS:

1. Preheat oven to 375°F.
2. In a bowl, combine chickpeas, broccoli, rice, yogurt, garlic, and seasoning.
3. Spread into a greased baking dish and top with cheese.
4. Bake for 20–25 minutes until hot and bubbly.
5. Let cool slightly before serving.

Nutrition:

Calories: 270 | **Protein:** 13g | **Fat:** 11g | **Carbohydrates:** 28g | **Fiber:** 6g

Tuna & White Bean Casserole

Prep Time: 20 minutes

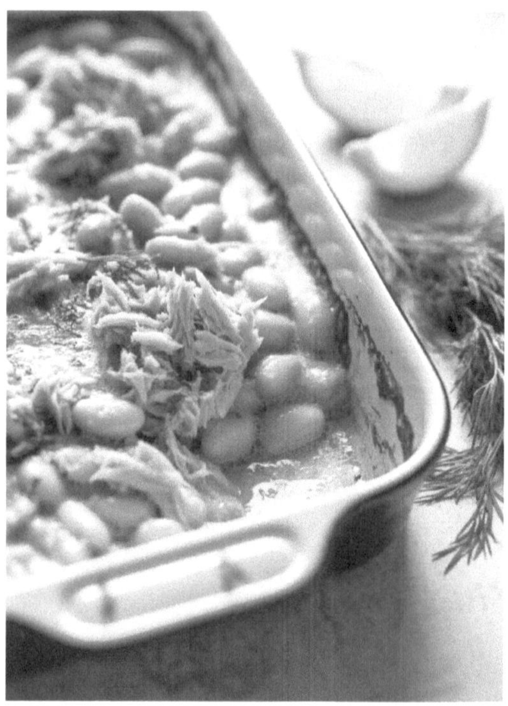

INGREDIENTS:

- 1 can tuna in water, drained
- 1 cup canned white beans, rinsed
- 1/2 cup cooked whole-grain pasta

- 1/4 cup plain Greek yogurt
- 1/4 cup diced celery
- 1 tbsp olive oil
- 1/4 tsp dill
- Salt and pepper to taste

INSTRUCTIONS:

1. Preheat oven to 375°F.
2. In a large bowl, mix tuna, beans, pasta, yogurt, celery, dill, salt, and pepper.
3. Spread mixture into a greased baking dish.
4. Bake uncovered for 20–25 minutes until heated through.
5. Serve warm.

Nutrition:

Calories: 290 | **Protein:** 20g | **Fat:** 9g | **Carbohydrates:** 30g | **Fiber:** 5g

Cauliflower & Lentil Brain Bake

Prep Time: 25 minutes

Serves: 4

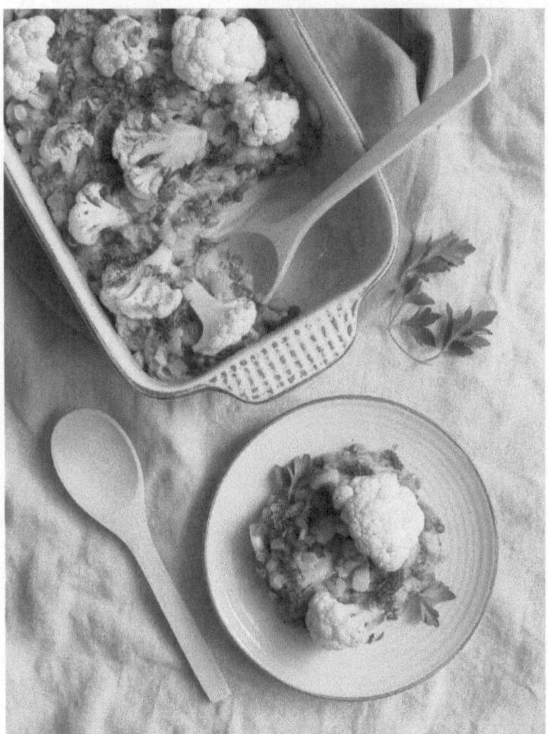

INGREDIENTS:

- 1 cup cooked lentils
- 2 cups chopped cauliflower florets
- 1/4 cup diced red onion
- 1/4 cup chopped parsley
- 1/4 cup shredded cheese or nutritional yeast
- 2 eggs
- 1/4 cup milk
- 1 tbsp olive oil
- Salt and pepper to taste

INSTRUCTIONS:

1. Preheat oven to 375°F.
2. Lightly steam cauliflower for 5 minutes.
3. In a bowl, combine lentils, cauliflower, onion, parsley, cheese, eggs, milk, and seasoning.
4. Pour into a greased baking dish and bake for 25–30 minutes.
5. Let cool slightly before serving.

Nutrition:

Calories: 240 | **Protein:** 14g | **Fat:** 10g | **Carbohydrates:** 22g | **Fiber:** 6g

PART 5: SNACKS, SIDES & SIPS

31. BRAIN-BOOSTING SNACKS

Walnut & Berry Trail Mix

Prep Time: 5 minutes

Serves: 4 (1/4 cup each)

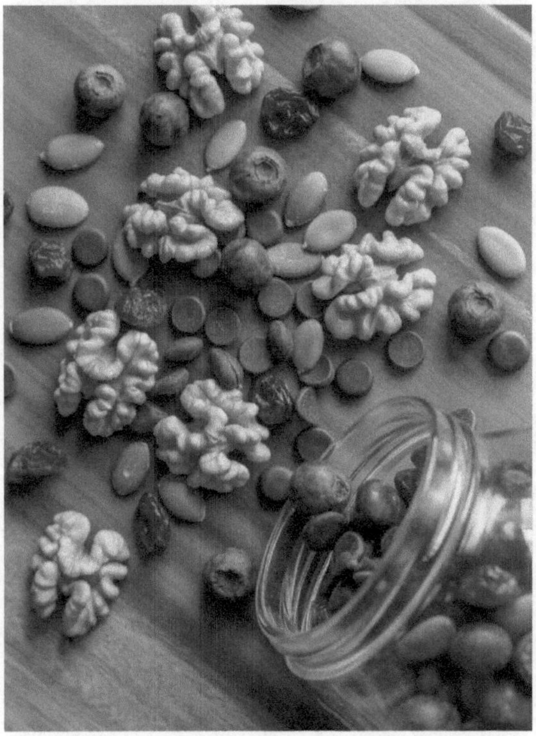

INGREDIENTS:

- 1/2 cup raw walnuts
- 1/4 cup dried cranberries (unsweetened)
- 1/4 cup dried blueberries
- 2 tbsp pumpkin seeds
- 1 tbsp dark chocolate chips (optional)

INSTRUCTIONS:

1. Combine all ingredients in a bowl and mix well.
2. Store in an airtight container for up to one week.
3. Enjoy as a grab-and-go brain-boosting snack.

Nutrition:

Calories: 180 | **Protein:** 4g | **Fat:** 15g | **Carbohydrates:** 12g | **Fiber:** 3g

Frozen Blueberry Yogurt Bites

Prep Time: 10 minutes (+2 hours freeze time)

Serves: 4

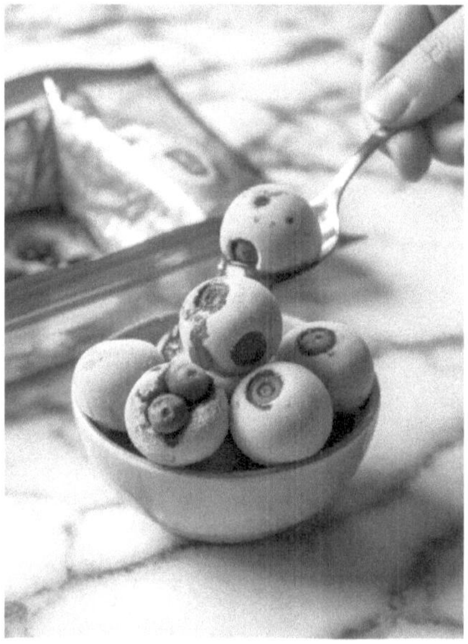

INGREDIENTS:

- 1/2 cup fresh blueberries
- 1/2 cup plain Greek yogurt
- 1 tsp honey (optional)

INSTRUCTIONS:

1. Line a small tray with parchment paper.
2. Dip each blueberry in yogurt and place on the tray.
3. Drizzle with honey if using.
4. Freeze for 2 hours until firm.
5. Store in a freezer-safe bag and enjoy cold.

Nutrition:

Calories: 90 | **Protein:** 5g | **Fat:** 2g | **Carbohydrates:** 12g | **Fiber:** 2g

Chia Almond Energy Balls

Prep Time: 15 minutes (no bake)

Serves: 6 (2 balls each)

INGREDIENTS:

- 1/2 cup rolled oats

- 1/4 cup almond butter
- 1 tbsp chia seeds
- 2 tbsp honey
- 1/4 cup chopped almonds
- 1/2 tsp cinnamon

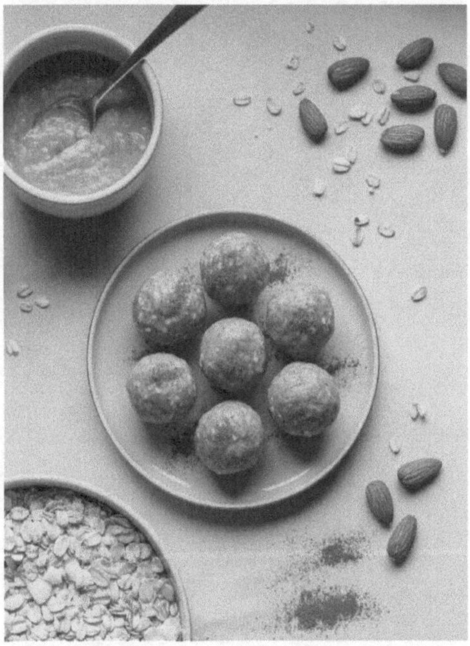

INSTRUCTIONS:

1. Mix all ingredients in a bowl until well combined.
2. Roll into small balls using your hands.
3. Place on a plate and refrigerate for at least 30 minutes.
4. Store in a sealed container for up to 5 days.

Nutrition:

Calories: 120 (per 2 balls) | **Protein:** 4g | **Fat:** 8g | **Carbohydrates:** 10g | **Fiber:** 2g |

Spiced Pumpkin Seed Crunch

Prep Time: 10 minutes

Serves: 4

INGREDIENTS:

- 1/2 cup raw pumpkin seeds
- 1/2 tsp olive oil

- 1/4 tsp paprika
- 1/4 tsp cinnamon
- Pinch of sea salt

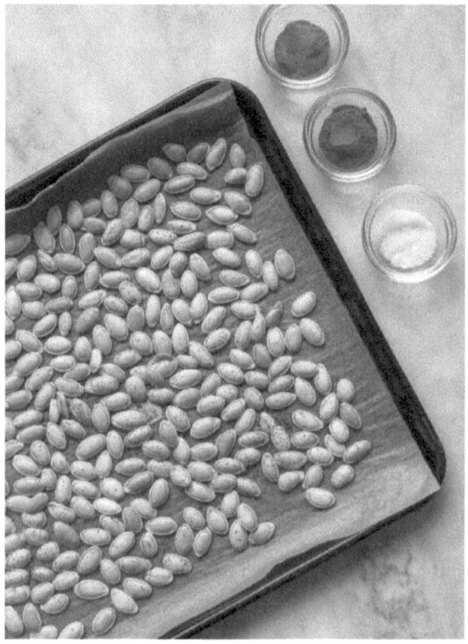

INSTRUCTIONS:

1. Preheat oven to 325°F.
2. Toss pumpkin seeds with olive oil, spices, and salt.
3. Spread on a baking sheet in a single layer.
4. Roast for 8–10 minutes, stirring halfway through.
5. Let cool before eating or storing.

Nutrition:

Calories: 130 | **Protein:** 6g | **Fat:** 11g | **Carbohydrates:** 4g | **Fiber:** 1g

Dark Chocolate Nut Clusters

Prep Time: 10 minutes (+15 minutes chill time)

Serves: 6

INGREDIENTS:

- 1/2 cup mixed nuts (walnuts, almonds, pistachios)
- 1/4 cup dark chocolate chips (70% or higher)
- Pinch of sea salt (optional)

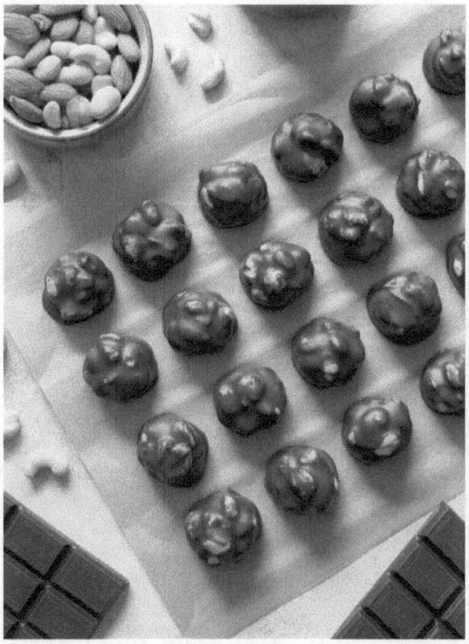

INSTRUCTIONS:

1. Melt chocolate chips in a microwave-safe bowl in 30-second intervals, stirring each time.
2. Mix in the nuts until fully coated.
3. Drop spoonfuls onto parchment paper.
4. Sprinkle with sea salt if desired.
5. Chill in the fridge for 15 minutes until firm.

Nutrition:

Calories: 160 | **Protein:** 4g | **Fat:** 13g | **Carbohydrates:** 8g | **Fiber:** 2g

32. VEGGIE-BASED DIPS & SPREADS

Roasted Red Pepper Hummus

Prep Time: 10 minutes

Serves: 6

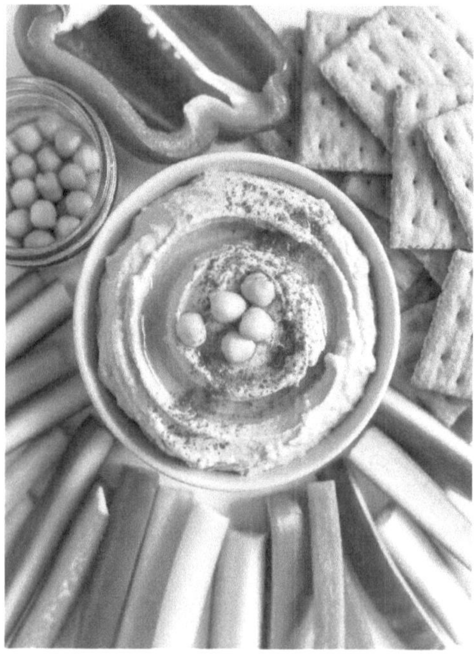

INGREDIENTS:

- 1 cup canned chickpeas, rinsed
- 1/2 cup roasted red peppers
- 2 tbsp tahini
- 1 tbsp olive oil
- 1 tbsp lemon juice
- 1 garlic clove
- Salt and pepper to taste

INSTRUCTIONS:

1. Combine all ingredients in a food processor or blender.
2. Blend until smooth, adding water if needed for texture.
3. Transfer to a bowl and serve with veggie sticks or whole-grain crackers.

Nutrition:

Calories: 100 | **Protein:** 3g | **Fat:** 6g | **Carbohydrates:** 9g | **Fiber:** 2g

Spinach & White Bean Spread

Prep Time: 10 minutes

Serves: 4

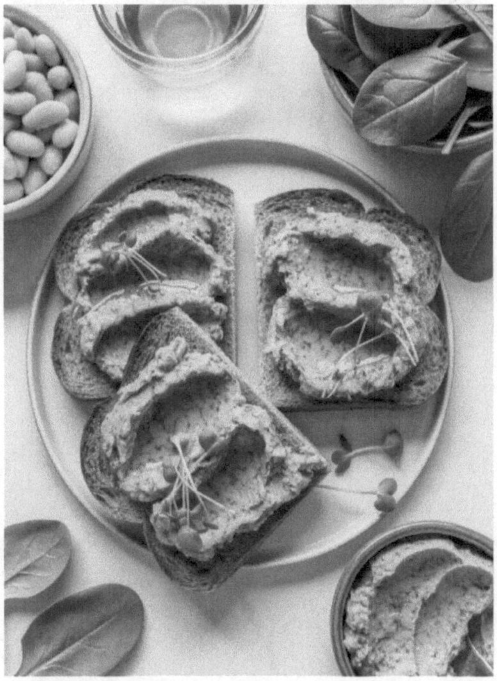

INGREDIENTS:

- 1/2 cup white beans (cooked or canned, rinsed)
- 1 cup fresh spinach, lightly steamed
- 1 tbsp olive oil
- 1 tbsp lemon juice
- 1 garlic clove
- Salt and pepper to taste

INSTRUCTIONS:

1. Place all ingredients in a blender or food processor.
2. Blend until creamy, scraping down sides as needed.
3. Serve with toast, crackers, or use as a sandwich spread.

Nutrition:

Calories: 90 | **Protein:** 4g | **Fat:** 5g | **Carbohydrates:** 8g | **Fiber:** 2g

Carrot & Ginger Dip

Prep Time: 15 minutes

Serves: 5

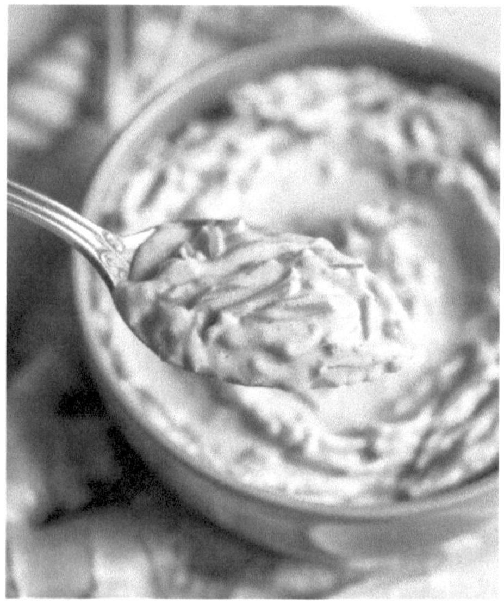

INGREDIENTS:

- 1 1/2 cups chopped carrots, steamed until soft
- 1 tbsp olive oil
- 1 tsp grated fresh ginger
- 1 tbsp lemon juice
- Salt and pepper to taste

INSTRUCTIONS:

1. Combine all ingredients in a food processor.
2. Blend until smooth and creamy.
3. Chill for 15 minutes before serving for best flavor.

Nutrition:

Calories: 80 | **Protein:** 1g | **Fat:** 4g | **Carbohydrates:** 10g | **Fiber:** 3g

Avocado Edamame Smash

Prep Time: 10 minutes

Serves: 4

INGREDIENTS:

- 1/2 ripe avocado

- 1/2 cup shelled edamame, cooked
- 1 tbsp lime juice
- 1 tbsp olive oil
- Salt and pepper to taste

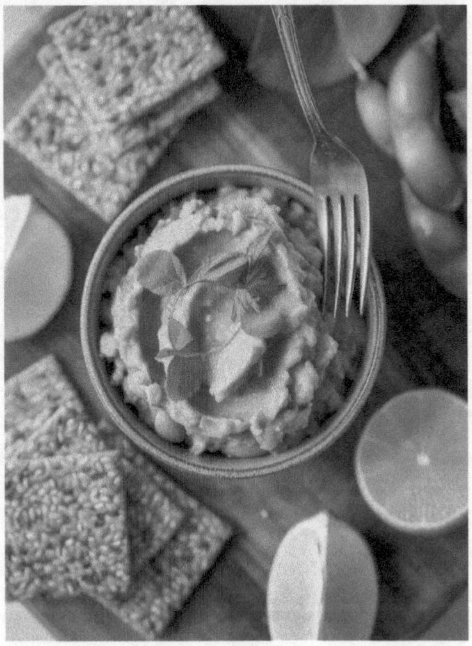

INSTRUCTIONS:

1. In a bowl, mash avocado and edamame together using a fork.
2. Stir in lime juice, olive oil, salt, and pepper.
3. Serve immediately as a dip or sandwich spread.

Nutrition:

Calories: 120 | **Protein:** 5g | **Fat:** 9g | **Carbohydrates:** 8g | **Fiber:** 4g

Beet & Yogurt Brain Dip

Prep Time: 10 minutes

Serves: 4

INGREDIENTS:

- 1 small roasted beet, peeled and chopped
- 1/2 cup plain Greek yogurt
- 1 tbsp lemon juice
- 1 garlic clove, minced

- Salt and pepper to taste

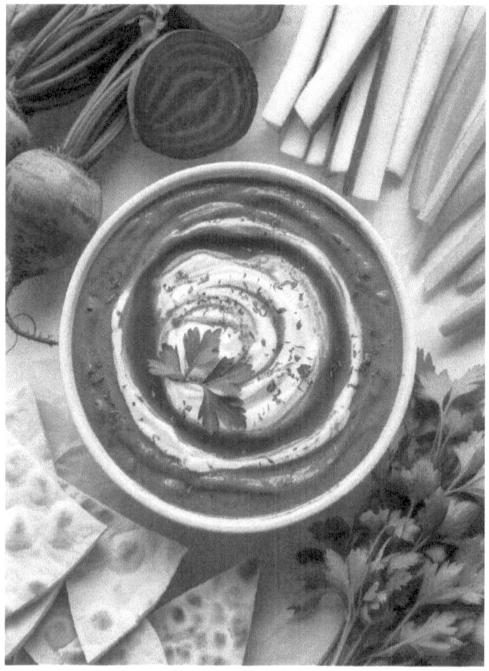

INSTRUCTIONS:

1. Place all ingredients in a blender or food processor.
2. Blend until smooth and vibrantly pink.
3. Chill before serving with raw veggies or pita wedges.

Nutrition:

Calories: 85 | **Protein:** 5g | **Fat:** 2g | **Carbohydrates:** 10g | **Fiber:** 2g

33. MOOD-SUPPORTING SOUPS & SIDES

Lentil & Turmeric Soup

Prep Time: 30 minutes

Serves: 4

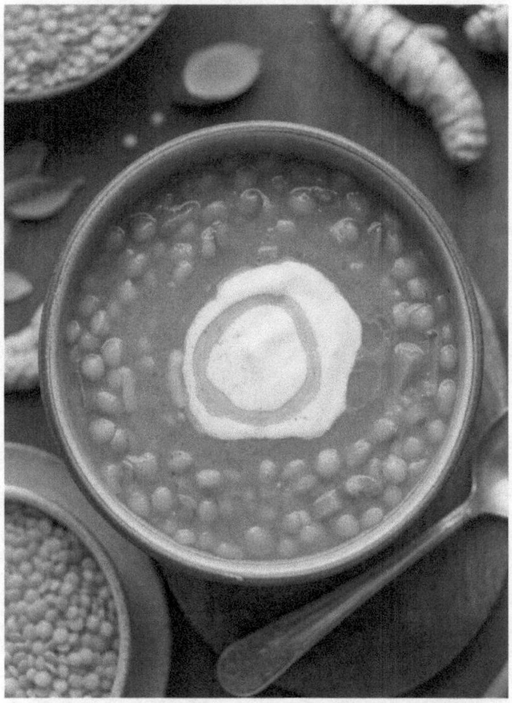

INGREDIENTS:

- 1 cup dried red lentils, rinsed
- 1/2 cup diced carrots
- 1/2 cup chopped onion
- 2 garlic cloves, minced
- 1 tsp ground turmeric
- 1 tbsp olive oil
- 4 cups low-sodium vegetable broth
- Salt and pepper to taste

INSTRUCTIONS:

1. In a pot, heat olive oil over medium heat. Sauté onions, garlic, and carrots for 5 minutes.
2. Stir in lentils and turmeric, then add broth.
3. Bring to a boil, then reduce heat and simmer for 20 minutes.
4. Season with salt and pepper, then serve warm.

Nutrition:

Calories: 210 | **Protein:** 13g | **Fat:** 6g | **Carbohydrates:** 27g | **Fiber:** 8g

Sweet Potato & Kale Mash

Prep Time: 25 minutes

Serves: 3

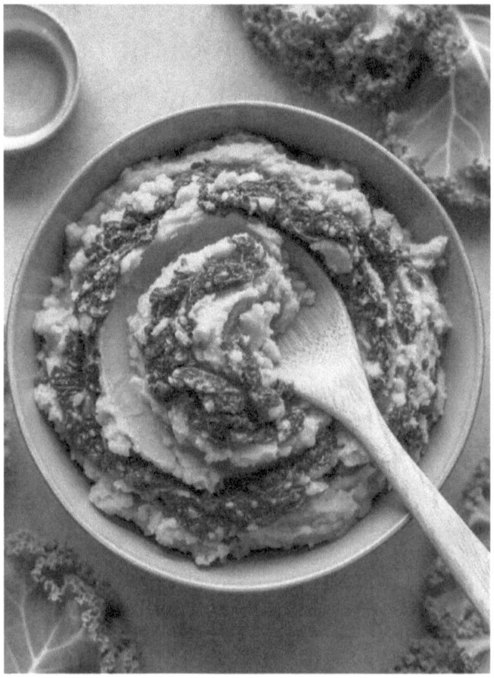

INGREDIENTS:

- 2 medium sweet potatoes, peeled and chopped
- 1 cup kale, chopped
- 1 tbsp olive oil
- Salt and pepper to taste

INSTRUCTIONS:

1. Boil sweet potatoes in a pot until tender, about 12–15 minutes.
2. Steam or sauté kale until wilted.
3. Drain potatoes and mash with olive oil, salt, and pepper.
4. Stir in kale and mix well before serving.

Nutrition:

Calories: 190 | **Protein:** 3g | **Fat:** 7g | **Carbohydrates:** 30g | **Fiber:** 5g

Miso Mushroom Broth Bowl

Prep Time: 20 minutes

Serves: 2

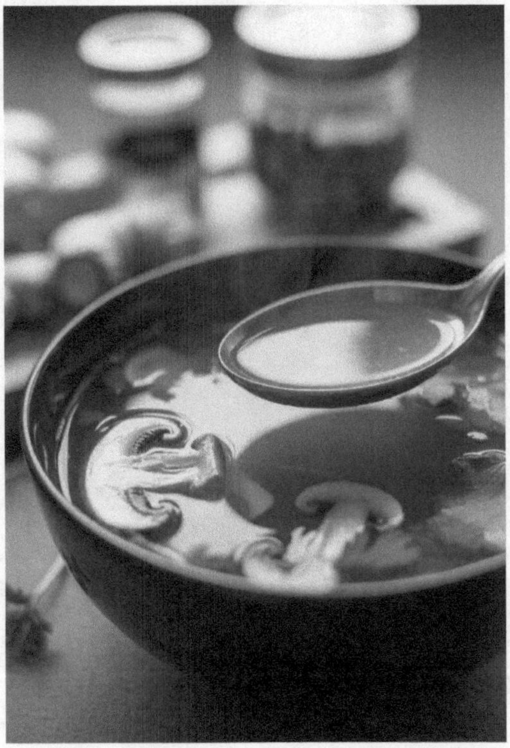

INGREDIENTS:

- 3 cups water
- 1 tbsp white miso paste
- 1/2 cup sliced mushrooms
- 1 green onion, chopped
- 1 tsp grated ginger
- 1/2 tsp sesame oil

INSTRUCTIONS:

1. In a pot, bring water to a light simmer.
2. Stir in miso paste until dissolved.
3. Add mushrooms, green onion, and ginger. Simmer for 10 minutes.
4. Drizzle with sesame oil and serve hot.

Nutrition:

Calories: 70 | **Protein:** 3g | **Fat:** 2g | **Carbohydrates:** 9g | **Fiber:** 1g

Roasted Carrot & Parsnip Wedges

Prep Time: 30 minutes

Serves: 4

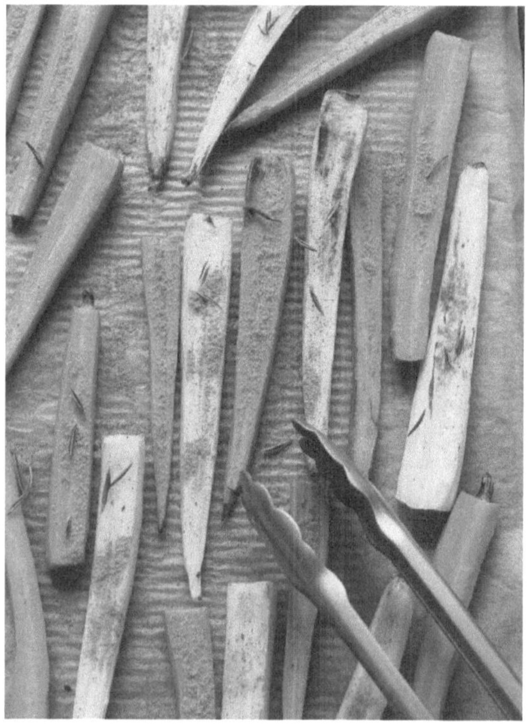

INGREDIENTS:

- 2 carrots, cut into sticks
- 2 parsnips, cut into sticks
- 1 tbsp olive oil
- 1/2 tsp cumin
- 1/4 tsp paprika
- Salt and pepper to taste

INSTRUCTIONS:

1. Preheat oven to 400°F.
2. Toss carrots and parsnips with olive oil and spices.
3. Spread on a baking sheet in a single layer.
4. Roast for 25 minutes, turning halfway through.
5. Serve warm as a side dish.

Nutrition:

Calories: 120 | **Protein:** 2g | **Fat:** 6g | **Carbohydrates:** 15g | **Fiber:** 4g

Cauliflower Tahini Mash

Prep Time: 20 minutes

Serves: 3

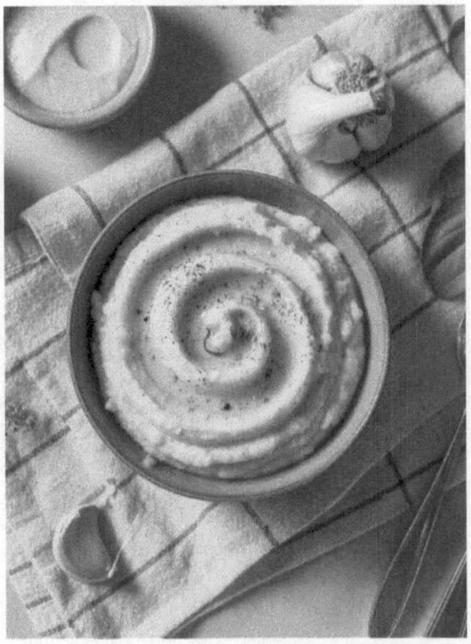

INGREDIENTS:

- 1 medium head cauliflower, cut into florets
- 1 tbsp tahini
- 1 tbsp olive oil
- 1 garlic clove, minced
- Salt and pepper to taste

INSTRUCTIONS:

1. Steam cauliflower until very soft, about 10 minutes.
2. In a food processor, blend cauliflower with tahini, olive oil, garlic, salt, and pepper until smooth.
3. Serve warm as a nourishing side or base for bowls.

Nutrition:

Calories: 130 | **Protein:** 4g | **Fat:** 10g | **Carbohydrates:** 9g | **Fiber:** 3g

34. HEALTHY FATS IN QUICK BITES

Avocado & Tuna Crispbreads

Prep Time: 10 minutes

Serves: 2

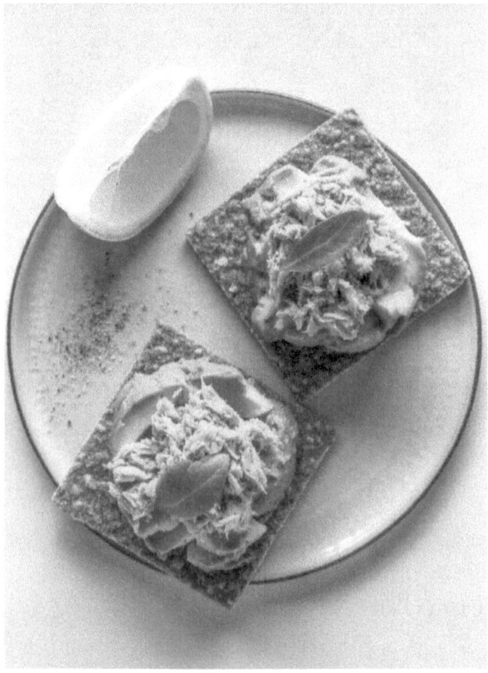

INGREDIENTS:

- 2 whole-grain crispbreads
- 1/2 avocado, mashed
- 1/2 can tuna in olive oil, drained
- Salt and pepper to taste
- Optional: squeeze of lemon juice

INSTRUCTIONS:

1. Spread mashed avocado on each crispbread.
2. Top with tuna and season with salt, pepper, and lemon juice if using.
3. Serve immediately for a light, satisfying snack.

Nutrition:

Calories: 240 | **Protein:** 14g | **Fat:** 16g | **Carbohydrates:** 10g | **Fiber:** 4g

Olive & Almond Snack Bowl

Prep Time: 2 minutes

Serves: 1

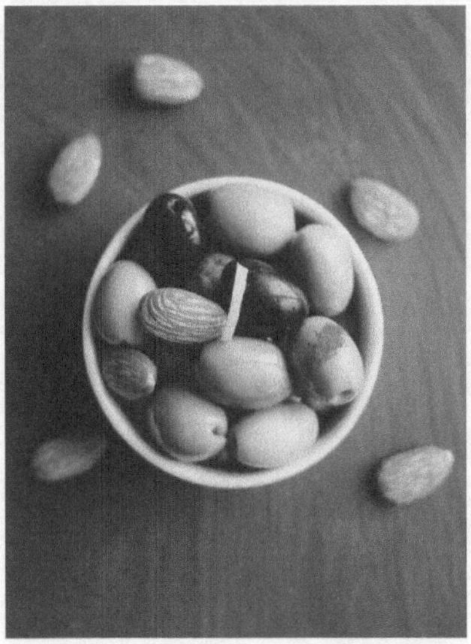

INGREDIENTS:

- 6–8 green or black olives
- 12 raw almonds
- Optional: sprinkle of paprika or lemon zest

INSTRUCTIONS:

1. Place olives and almonds in a small bowl.
2. Add paprika or lemon zest for extra flavor if desired.
3. Enjoy as a quick Mediterranean-inspired bite.

Nutrition:

Calories: 170 | **Protein:** 4g | **Fat:** 15g | **Carbohydrates:** 5g | **Fiber:** 3g

Mini Stuffed Avocado Boats

Prep Time: 10 minutes

Serves: 2

INGREDIENTS:

- 1 ripe avocado, halved and pitted
- 2 tbsp hummus
- 1 tbsp sunflower seeds

- Pinch of paprika

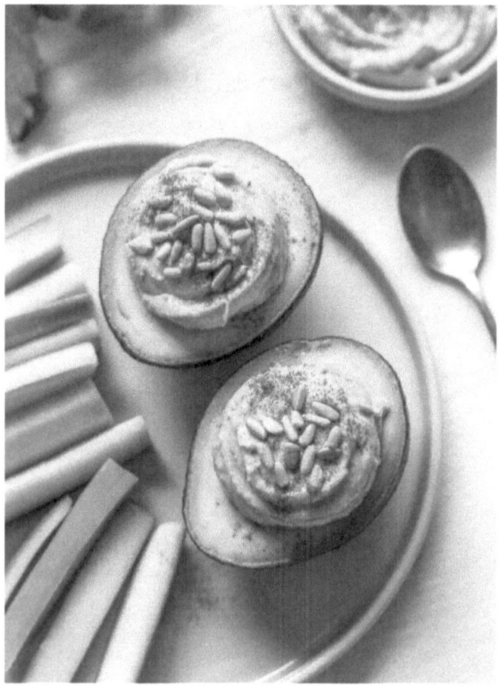

INSTRUCTIONS:

1. Fill each avocado half with 1 tablespoon of hummus.
2. Sprinkle with sunflower seeds and paprika.
3. Serve with a spoon or scoop with veggie sticks.

Nutrition:

Calories: 200 | **Protein:** 5g | **Fat:** 18g | **Carbohydrates:** 8g | **Fiber:** 6g

Smoked Salmon & Avocado Roll-Ups

Prep Time: 10 minutes

Serves: 2

INGREDIENTS:

- 2 slices smoked salmon
- 1/4 avocado, sliced thin
- 1 tsp cream cheese or hummus
- Fresh dill or arugula (optional)

INSTRUCTIONS:

1. Lay out smoked salmon slices on a plate.

2. Spread a thin layer of cream cheese or hummus.
3. Add avocado slices and herbs, then roll up.
4. Secure with toothpicks if needed and serve chilled.

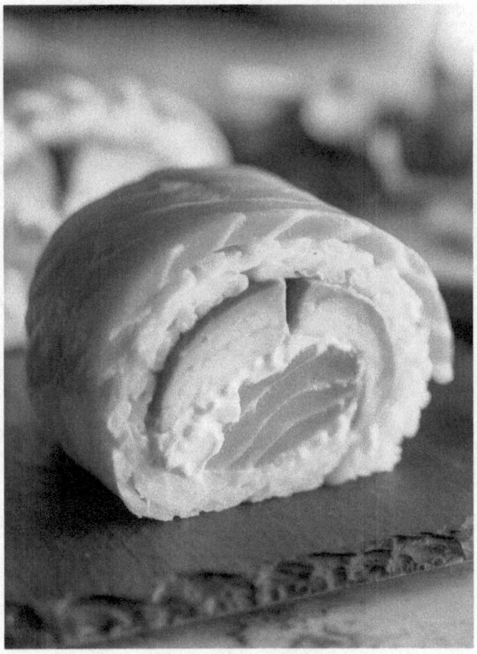

Nutrition:

Calories: 180 | **Protein:** 11g | **Fat:** 13g | **Carbohydrates:** 3g | **Omega-3s:** High | **Brain Support:** Moderate

Nutty Apple Rounds

Prep Time: 5 minutes

Serves: 2

INGREDIENTS:

- 1 medium apple, sliced into rings
- 2 tbsp almond or peanut butter
- 1 tbsp crushed walnuts or pistachios

INSTRUCTIONS:

1. Core the apple and slice it into round rings.
2. Spread nut butter over each slice.
3. Sprinkle with crushed nuts and serve immediately.

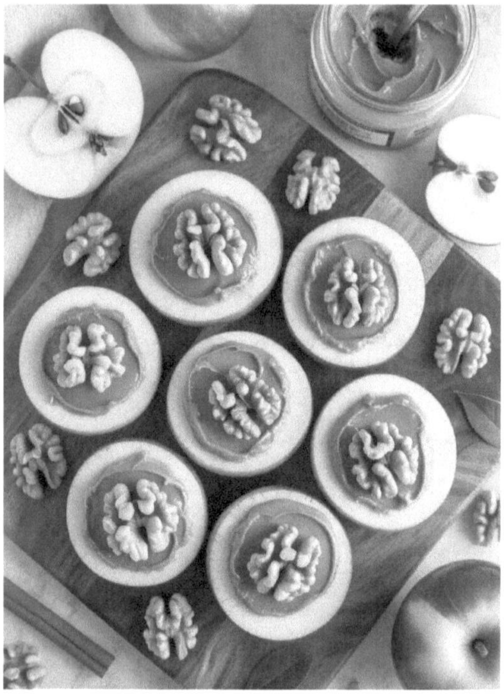

Nutrition:

Calories: 210 | **Protein:** 5g | **Fat:** 14g | **Carbohydrates:** 20g | **Fiber:** 4g

35. SMOOTHIES, JUICES & INFUSED WATERS

Cucumber Mint Infused Water

Prep Time: 5 minutes (+1 hour infusion)

Serves: 4

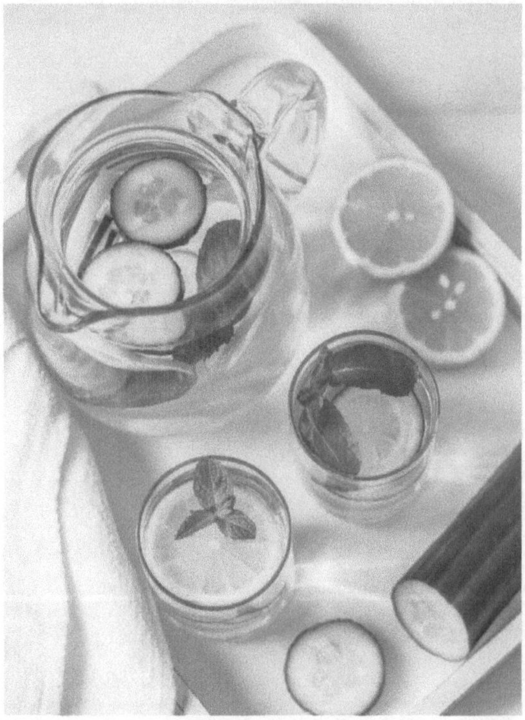

INGREDIENTS:

- 4 cups water
- 1/2 cucumber, thinly sliced
- 5–6 fresh mint leaves
- Optional: 2 lemon slices

INSTRUCTIONS:

1. Add cucumber, mint, and lemon to a pitcher of water.
2. Chill in the fridge for at least 1 hour before drinking.
3. Enjoy throughout the day for hydration and refreshment.

Nutrition:

Calories: 5 | **Protein:** 0g | **Fat:** 0g | **Carbohydrates:** 1g | **Fiber:** 0g

Orange Carrot Ginger Juice

Prep Time: 10 minutes

Serves: 2

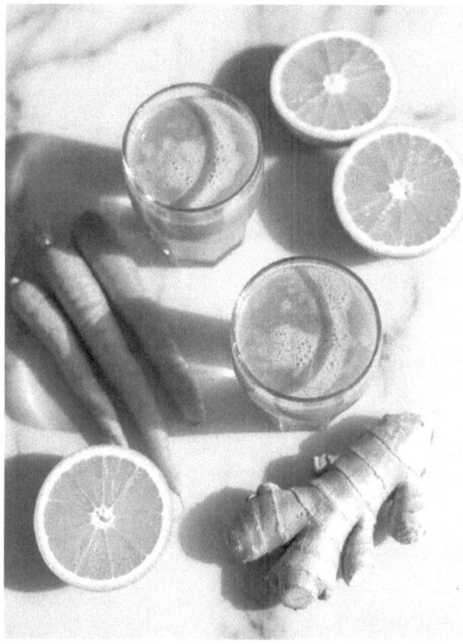

INGREDIENTS:

- 2 medium carrots, peeled
- 2 oranges, peeled
- 1/2 inch piece fresh ginger
- 1/2 cup water

INSTRUCTIONS:

1. Blend all ingredients in a high-speed blender until smooth.
2. Strain through a fine mesh or drink as-is for more fiber.
3. Serve chilled.

Nutrition:

Calories: 90 | **Protein:** 1g | **Fat:** 0g | **Carbohydrates:** 20g | **Fiber:** 3g

Green Focus Smoothie

Prep Time: 5 minutes

Serves: 1

INGREDIENTS:

- 1/2 banana

- 1/2 cup spinach
- 1/4 avocado
- 1/2 cup unsweetened almond milk
- 1 tbsp chia seeds

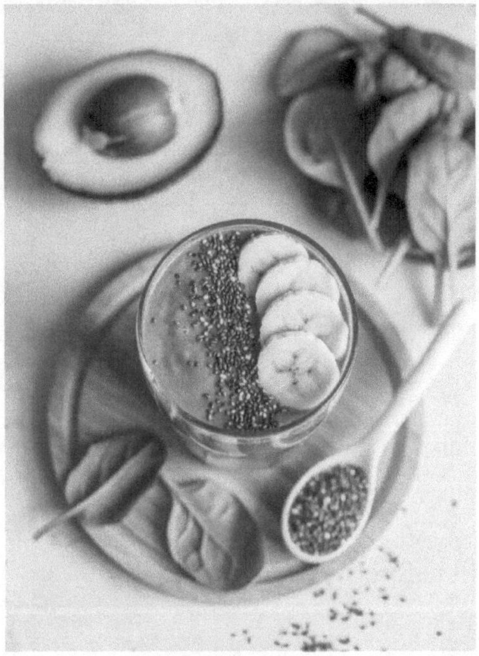

INSTRUCTIONS:

1. Add all ingredients to a blender.
2. Blend until creamy and smooth.
3. Pour into a glass and enjoy immediately.

Nutrition:

Calories: 190 | **Protein:** 4g | **Fat:** 12g | **Carbohydrates:** 16g | **Fiber:** 6g

Blueberry Basil Sparkling Water

Prep Time: 5 minutes (+15 minutes infusion)

Serves: 2

INGREDIENTS:

- 1/4 cup fresh blueberries
- 4 fresh basil leaves
- 2 cups sparkling water
- Ice (optional)

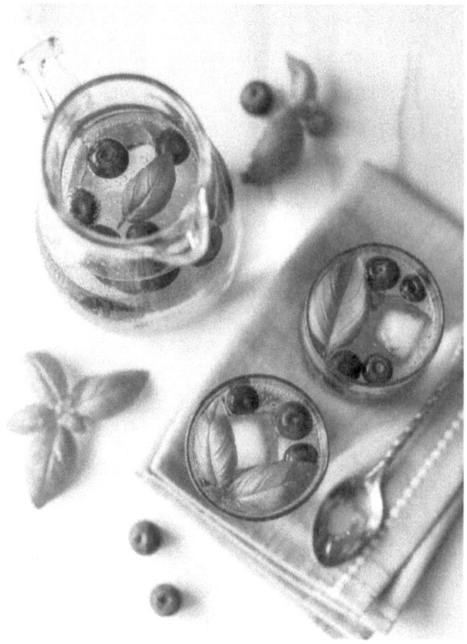

INSTRUCTIONS:

1. Gently muddle blueberries and basil in a glass or pitcher.
2. Add sparkling water and stir.
3. Let sit for 10–15 minutes or chill before serving over ice.

Nutrition:

Calories: 10 | **Protein:** 0g | **Fat:** 0g | **Carbohydrates:** 2g | **Fiber:** 0g

Beet & Berry Brain Smoothie

Prep Time: 5 minutes

Serves: 1

INGREDIENTS:

- 1/2 small cooked beet
- 1/2 cup frozen mixed berries
- 1/2 cup unsweetened almond milk
- 1 tbsp ground flaxseed
- 1/2 tsp cinnamon

INSTRUCTIONS:

1. Blend all ingredients until smooth and creamy.
2. Serve immediately.
3. Optionally top with a few fresh berries or chia seeds.

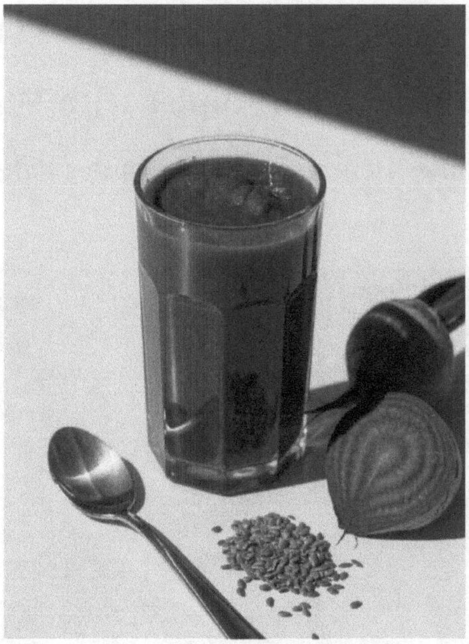

Nutrition:

Calories: 170 | **Protein:** 3g | **Fat:** 6g | **Carbohydrates:** 26g | **Fiber:** 5g | **Nitrates:** High | **Brain Antioxidants:** High

36. SWEET TREATS WITH MEMORY BENEFITS

Baked Cinnamon Apples with Walnuts

Prep Time: 10 minutes (+20 minutes bake time)

Serves: 2

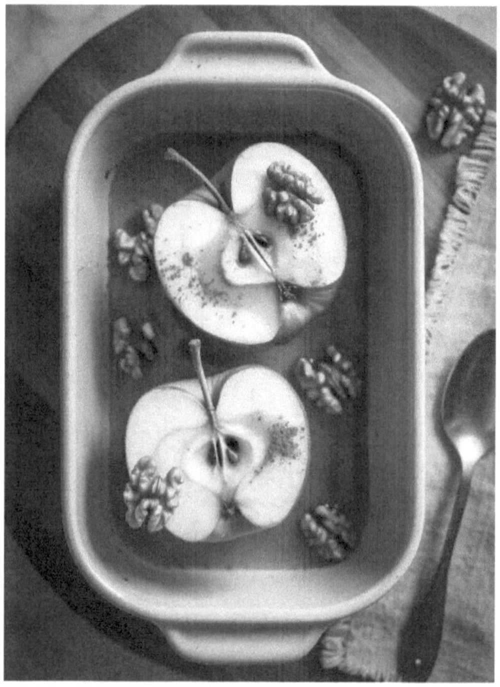

INGREDIENTS:

- 2 medium apples, cored and halved
- 2 tbsp chopped walnuts
- 1/2 tsp cinnamon
- 1 tsp maple syrup
- 1/2 tsp coconut oil

INSTRUCTIONS:

1. Preheat oven to 375°F.
2. Place apple halves in a baking dish and top with walnuts.
3. Sprinkle with cinnamon, drizzle with maple syrup, and dot with coconut oil.
4. Bake for 20 minutes until tender.
5. Serve warm.

Nutrition:

Calories: 180 | **Protein:** 2g | **Fat:** 9g | **Carbohydrates:** 24g | **Fiber:** 4g

Dark Chocolate Blueberry Bites

Prep Time: 5 minutes (+15 minutes chill time)

Serves: 4

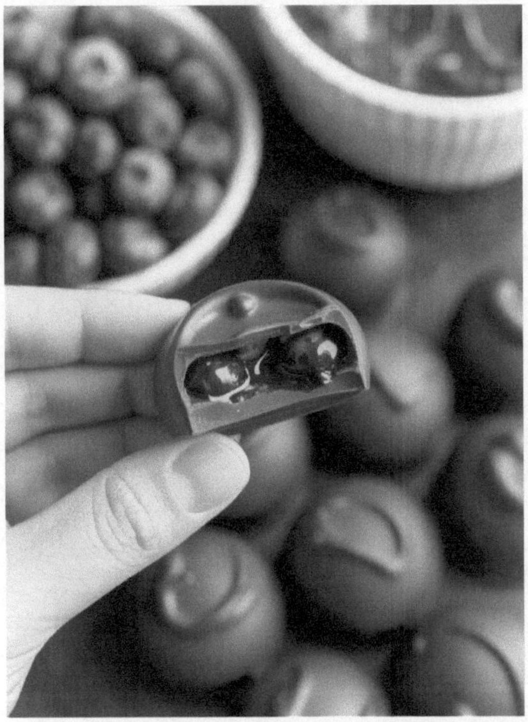

INGREDIENTS:

- 1/2 cup fresh blueberries
- 1/4 cup dark chocolate chips (70% or higher)

INSTRUCTIONS:

1. Melt chocolate chips in a microwave-safe bowl in 30-second intervals.
2. Spoon a few blueberries into mini muffin liners or onto parchment.
3. Drizzle with melted chocolate to coat.
4. Chill in the fridge for 15 minutes until set.
5. Serve cold.

Nutrition:

Calories: 130 | **Protein:** 1g | **Fat:** 8g | **Carbohydrates:** 14g | **Fiber:** 2g

Frozen Yogurt Berry Bark

Prep Time: 10 minutes (+2 hours freeze time)

Serves: 6

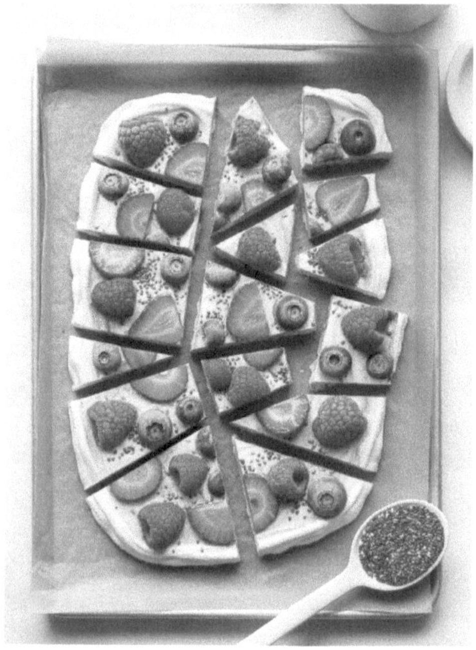

INGREDIENTS:

- 1 cup plain Greek yogurt
- 1/2 cup mixed berries
- 1 tbsp chia seeds
- 1 tsp honey (optional)

INSTRUCTIONS:

1. Spread yogurt onto a parchment-lined baking sheet.
2. Scatter berries and chia seeds over the top.
3. Drizzle with honey if using.
4. Freeze for at least 2 hours, then break into pieces.
5. Store in a freezer-safe bag.

Nutrition:

Calories: 90 | **Protein:** 6g | **Fat:** 2g | **Carbohydrates:** 12g | **Fiber:** 2g

Avocado Chocolate Pudding

Prep Time: 5 minutes

Serves: 2

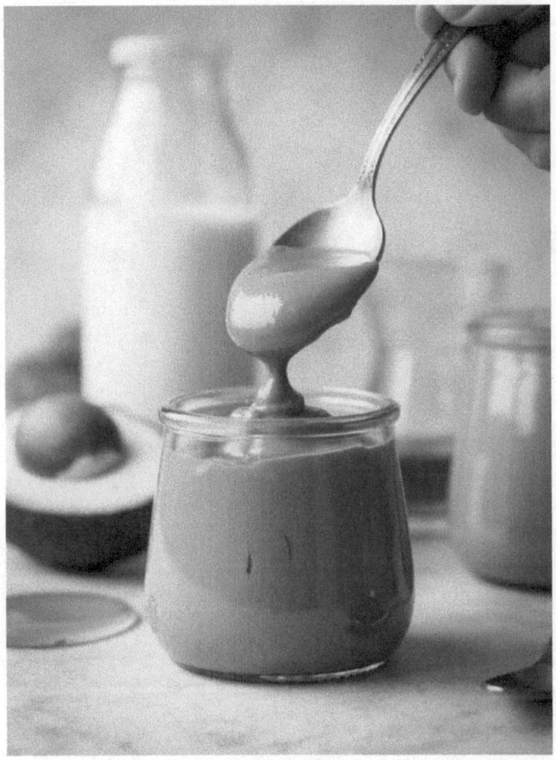

INGREDIENTS:

- 1 ripe avocado
- 2 tbsp unsweetened cocoa powder
- 2 tbsp maple syrup or honey
- 1/4 cup unsweetened almond milk
- 1/2 tsp vanilla extract

INSTRUCTIONS:

1. Blend all ingredients in a food processor until smooth.
2. Scrape down sides and blend again if needed.
3. Chill for 15 minutes before serving.

Nutrition:

Calories: 210 | **Protein:** 3g | **Fat:** 15g | **Carbohydrates:** 18g | **Fiber:** 5g

Oatmeal Raisin No-Bake Cookies

Prep Time: 10 minutes (+20 minutes chill time)

Serves: 6

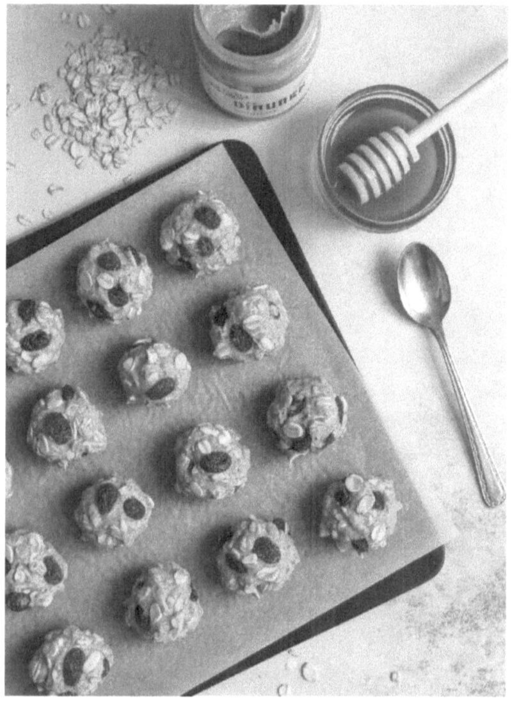

INGREDIENTS:

- 1/2 cup rolled oats
- 1/4 cup almond butter
- 1/4 cup raisins
- 1 tbsp flaxseed meal
- 1 tbsp honey or maple syrup
- 1/2 tsp cinnamon

INSTRUCTIONS:

1. Mix all ingredients in a bowl until well combined.
2. Scoop into small rounds and place on parchment paper.
3. Chill for 20 minutes to firm up.
4. Store in the fridge for up to 5 days.

Nutrition:

Calories: 120 | **Protein:** 3g | **Fat:** 6g | **Carbohydrates:** 15g | **Fiber:** 3g

PART 6:

LIFESTYLE & LONG-TERM VITALITY

37. STAYING MENTALLY SHARP BEYOND THE PLATE: DAILY ROUTINES FOR LONGEVITY & WELLNESS

Certainly! Below is a **700-word** section for **PART 6: Lifestyle & Long-Term Vitality**, titled **"37. Staying Mentally Sharp Beyond the Plate: Daily Routines for Longevity & Wellness"**, following all of your instructions:

- **No em dashes at all**
- Only periods, commas, question marks, and apostrophes
- Written in clear, encouraging language appropriate for seniors over 60

37. Staying Mentally Sharp Beyond the Plate: Daily Routines for Longevity & Wellness

Eating for brain health is essential, but food is only part of the picture. The choices we make every day, from how we move to how we sleep, play a huge role in staying mentally sharp. If you want to protect your memory, improve your focus, and stay independent for years to come, your daily habits matter more than you might think.

The good news is you do not need a perfect routine. You just need a steady one. When your days are filled with small, positive choices, they build up over time and support long-term wellness. These choices do not need to be complex or exhausting. In fact, the best habits are often simple and easy to stick with.

Let us start with **movement**. Regular physical activity helps boost blood flow to the brain. This means more oxygen, more nutrients, and better mental clarity. Even a daily walk around the neighborhood can support better memory and mood. You do not need to run marathons. Gentle stretching, chair yoga, gardening, or dancing in the kitchen all count. Try to move your body for at least 30 minutes a day. Break it into two or three shorter sessions if that feels easier.

Sleep is another major factor in mental sharpness. Your brain uses sleep to clean out waste, form new memories, and reset your mood. Poor sleep can leave you foggy, irritable, and more likely to forget things. To sleep better, aim to go to bed and wake up at the same time each day. Turn off screens an hour before bed, keep your bedroom cool and quiet, and avoid caffeine in the afternoon. A short nap can be helpful too, as long as it does not interfere with nighttime sleep.

Mental activity matters just as much as physical activity. Just like your muscles, your brain needs regular use to stay strong. Keep your mind engaged with puzzles, reading, journaling, or learning something new. Try crosswords, Sudoku, or even a new language. Take up painting, writing, or playing an instrument. These creative tasks not only exercise your brain but also help relieve stress and boost mood.

Social connection is a powerful tool for brain health. Seniors who stay socially active tend to have sharper minds and better emotional health. Call a friend. Join a book club. Attend a community class or volunteer. Even short conversations can lift your spirits and keep your brain engaged. If in-person meetups are hard, try video calls or letter writing. Relationships are nourishment for the mind.

Another routine to support mental wellness is **managing stress**. Chronic stress affects memory, focus, and decision-making. It can also increase inflammation, which harms both brain and heart health. Use relaxation techniques like deep breathing, meditation, prayer, or quiet time in nature. Even five minutes of stillness each day can calm the nervous system. Try keeping a gratitude journal. Each morning, write down one thing you are thankful for. It is a simple act that trains your brain to notice the positive.

Hydration is easy to overlook but incredibly important. Even mild dehydration can affect concentration and memory. Aim for six to eight cups of water a day. If plain water feels boring, try herbal teas or infuse your water with fruit or cucumber slices. If you take medications, ask your doctor how much fluid you should be drinking.

Routine and structure can also support mental clarity. A predictable daily rhythm helps your brain stay organized and less stressed. Wake up and eat meals around the same time each day. Set simple goals. Prepare things the night before. Keep a calendar or use reminders to stay on track. When your days are calm and consistent, your mind works better.

Finally, do not underestimate the power of **purpose**. Having a reason to get up in the morning keeps your brain active and your heart full. That purpose might be taking care of a pet, tending a garden, helping grandchildren, or working on a creative project. Whatever brings you meaning is worth doing regularly. Purpose supports not just mental clarity but also emotional well-being and longevity.

These daily habits are not about being perfect. They are about building a life that supports your brain, your body, and your spirit. When you combine a brain-healthy diet with physical movement, mental engagement, sleep, connection, and calm, you give yourself the best possible chance for a long and vibrant life.

So move a little, laugh a little, rest deeply, and keep learning. The choices you make today shape the strength of your mind tomorrow. Your brain is worth the care.

38. GLOSSARY OF INGREDIENTS & NUTRITIONAL TERMS

38. Glossary of Ingredients & Nutritional Terms

1. Antioxidants

Compounds that protect cells from damage caused by free radicals and support brain and heart health.

2. Omega-3 Fatty Acids

Healthy fats found in fish, walnuts, and flaxseeds that reduce inflammation and support memory and focus.

3. Fiber

A plant-based nutrient that aids digestion, stabilizes blood sugar, and supports heart and brain health.

4. Whole Grains

Grains like brown rice, oats, and quinoa that contain all parts of the grain and more nutrients.

5. Folate

A B vitamin found in leafy greens and beans that supports mood, memory, and brain development.

6. Choline

A nutrient in eggs and broccoli important for memory and brain cell communication.

7. Probiotics

Live bacteria found in yogurt and fermented foods that support gut and brain health.

8. Flavonoids

Natural compounds in berries and dark chocolate that help protect the brain from aging.

9. Saturated Fat

A type of fat found in butter and fatty meats that can increase heart and brain risk if overconsumed.

10. Monounsaturated Fat

Healthy fat in olive oil, nuts, and avocados that supports blood flow and cognitive health.

11. Plant Protein

Protein from beans, lentils, and seeds that supports muscle and brain function without added fat.

12. Vitamin B12

A vitamin found in animal products that helps make red blood cells and maintain brain function.

13. Magnesium

A mineral that supports muscle relaxation, sleep, and memory. Found in leafy greens and seeds.

14. Iron

A mineral that helps carry oxygen in the blood and supports energy and concentration.

15. Nitrates

Compounds in beets and leafy greens that improve blood flow to the brain and heart.

16. Turmeric

A spice rich in curcumin, known for its anti-inflammatory and memory-supporting properties.

17. Glycemic Index

A scale that measures how quickly foods raise blood sugar levels after eating.

18. Legumes

Beans, lentils, and peas rich in fiber, protein, and brain-supporting nutrients.

19. Hydration

The process of keeping the body supplied with enough water to support focus and physical function.

20. Vitamin D

A nutrient that supports bone and brain health, often absorbed through sunlight or found in fish and eggs.

39. FAQS ON SENIOR NUTRITION

What makes senior nutrition different from younger adults?

As we age, our bodies change in many ways. We often need fewer calories but more nutrients. Our metabolism slows down, muscle mass may decrease, and digestion can become more sensitive. Seniors need more calcium, vitamin D, fiber, and protein to support bone health, brain function, and heart wellness. Hydration also becomes more important. Eating less does not mean eating poorly. In fact, every bite counts more than ever.

Is it really that important to limit sodium?

Yes, it is. Too much sodium can raise blood pressure, which increases the risk of heart disease and stroke. High blood pressure also affects blood flow to the brain, which may impact memory and focus. Many processed foods are full of hidden salt. Choosing fresh or minimally processed foods helps reduce sodium intake. Seasoning meals with herbs, lemon juice, and spices instead of salt can keep meals flavorful without the risks.

Can I still eat carbohydrates on a brain-healthy diet?

Absolutely. Carbohydrates are not the enemy, but it is important to choose the right kind. Whole grains like oats, brown rice, and quinoa provide long-lasting energy, fiber, and key nutrients. They help regulate blood sugar and keep the brain fueled. What seniors should avoid are refined carbs like white bread, pastries, and sugary snacks. These spike blood sugar and offer little nutritional value. Choosing complex carbs keeps energy steady and supports focus.

How much protein do older adults need?

Many seniors do not get enough protein, especially those who eat less or have dental concerns. Protein helps preserve muscle mass, supports immune function, and aids in healing. Good sources include eggs, fish, poultry, beans, lentils, tofu, nuts, and dairy. Aim to include some form of protein with every meal or snack. Even small servings, spread throughout the day, can make a big difference in strength and vitality.

Are plant-based diets safe and effective for seniors?

Yes, they can be very beneficial. Plant-based diets emphasize whole foods, fiber, antioxidants, and healthy fats, all of which support heart and brain health. Seniors who choose plant-based eating should ensure they get enough vitamin B12, calcium, iron, and protein. These can be found in fortified foods or with guidance from a healthcare provider. Many seniors thrive on a mostly plant-based diet, especially when meals are balanced and varied.

What are the best foods to support memory and focus?

Some of the top brain-boosting foods include leafy greens, berries, walnuts, fatty fish like salmon, olive oil, beans, and whole grains. These foods reduce inflammation, support blood flow, and protect brain cells. They are rich in nutrients like omega-3s, antioxidants, B vitamins, and fiber. Including a variety of these foods throughout the week can help improve cognitive function, stabilize mood, and protect against age-related decline.

How can I make healthy meals without spending a lot of time or money?

Healthy eating does not have to be complicated or expensive. Start with simple recipes that use five ingredients or fewer. Buy produce that is in season or frozen, as both are often more affordable. Canned beans, whole grains, and eggs are cost-effective and nutrient-rich. Batch cooking and using leftovers wisely can also save time and reduce waste. Planning meals ahead helps you avoid last-minute takeout and ensures you get the nutrients your body needs.

What are some tips for eating well if I live alone or have little appetite?

Seniors who live alone often skip meals or fall into repetitive eating habits. Try to create small routines around mealtime, even if you are the only one at the table. Set the table, play music, or eat near a sunny window. Choose smaller, nutrient-dense meals if your appetite is low. Smoothies, soups, and small bowls of grains, greens, and protein can go a long way. Invite a friend to share a meal once a week or connect with community programs that offer shared dining or meal delivery.

Do supplements replace the need for healthy food?

Supplements can be helpful in certain cases, especially if your doctor identifies a deficiency. But they are not a substitute for a healthy diet. Whole foods contain a wide range of nutrients that work together to support your health in ways that isolated pills cannot. If you are concerned about vitamin D, B12, or calcium, talk to your healthcare provider about what supplements may help. Otherwise, aim to get most of your nutrients from real food. A colorful plate is often the best form of prevention and protection.

40. FINAL THOUGHTS: A LONG, SHARP, INDEPENDENT LIFE

Aging is not something to fear. It is a chapter filled with wisdom, perspective, and possibility. While it may bring certain changes, it also brings the opportunity to take control of your health in a powerful and lasting way.

Throughout this book, you have learned how nutrition directly supports the brain and body. You have seen how simple foods like leafy greens, berries, olive oil, and whole grains can do more than fill a plate. They protect memory, improve focus, boost mood, and help prevent decline. You have explored how movement, sleep, hydration, and purpose can work together with food to keep your mind clear and your body strong.

The goal is not perfection. The goal is progress. Every small choice matters. Whether you prepare a five-ingredient meal, go for a walk, or spend a few quiet minutes in reflection, you are sending a message to your body and mind. That message is: I am worth taking care of.

You have the ability to shape your future with the choices you make today. You can enjoy your meals, move with purpose, connect with others, and stay sharp through the decades. Healthy aging is not about strict rules. It is about building habits that support who you are and how you want to live.

Let this be your new beginning. One rooted in strength, clarity, and confidence. You deserve a life filled with joy, independence, and sharp thinking.

Your brain is powerful. Feed it well, care for it daily, and trust it to carry you forward. The best years can still be ahead. Let them be bright. Let them be strong. Let them be yours.